Everyday diabetic

Publications International, Ltd.

Pictured on the front cover: (*clockwise from top left*): Thai Grilled Chicken (*page 108*), Fast Guacamole (*page 166*), Fruit Salad (*page 176*), and Roasted Chicken Salad (*page 54*).

Pictured on the back cover (*clockwise from top left*): Breakfast Quinoa (*page 13*), Couscous and Vegetable Risotto (*page 130*), Provençal Lemon and Olive Chicken (*page 118*), Creamy Coleslaw (*page 125*), Quinoa Burrito Bowls (*page 36*), and Peach-Melba Shortcakes (*page 173*).

Photographs on front cover and *page 54* copyright © Shutterstock.com.

ISBN: 978-1-64558-208-3

Manufactured in China.

8 7 6 5 4 3 2 1

Microwave Cooking: Microwave ovens vary in wattage. Use the cooking times as guidelines and check for doneness before adding more time.

Let's get social!

@Publications_International

@PublicationsInternational

www.pilcookbooks.com

contents

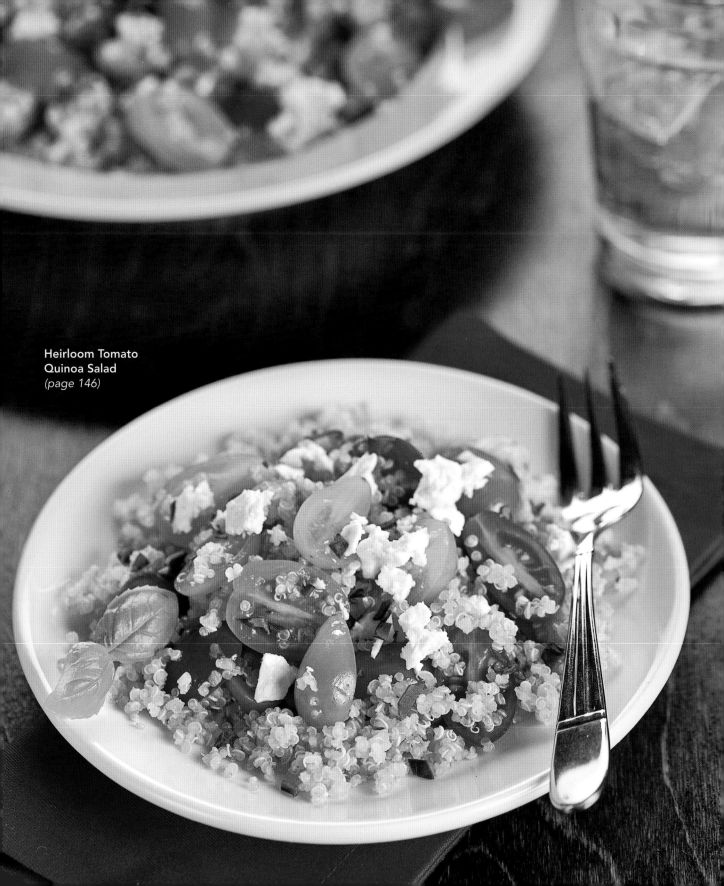

**Heirloom Tomato
Quinoa Salad**
(page 146)

introduction

WHAT IS DIABETES?

Millions of people today either may have diabetes or are at risk for getting diabetes. Although there is currently no cure for the disease, it is very treatable. You can easily live a long and healthy life by understanding diabetes and taking care of yourself.

To get the most from the latest advances in diabetes care, you need to understand just what it means to have diabetes. A good place to start is learning how the body uses fuel and how that process goes awry in diabetes.

EDUCATING YOURSELF

Even if you've only recently been diagnosed with diabetes, you've probably already heard the word glucose. It's an important player in the body and in diabetes. In your bloodstream, circulating to all your body parts, is sugar.

Most of the sugar in your bloodstream is the kind called glucose. Glucose's main job is to supply the body's cells with energy. Glucose is a quickly available fuel used by nearly all tissues in the body, and it's the only fuel your brain and nerves can use. The brain can survive without glucose for only a short time. Therefore, your brain directs your body to protect your glucose level, making sure it doesn't fall too low. It does this by increasing the production of certain hormones. These hormones cause the liver to release its stored-up sugar into the bloodstream. So, when people talk about blood sugar, they are really talking about glucose.

The glucose in your body comes from three major nutrients: fat, protein, and carbohydrate. About 10 percent of the fat and 50 percent of the protein you eat is eventually converted into glucose (the rest is used for other purposes or stored in

GLUCOSE

Most of the sugar in your bloodstream is the kind called glucose. Glucose's main job is to supply the body's cells with energy. It's a quickly available fuel used by nearly all tissues in the body, and it's the only fuel your brain and nerves can use.

INSULIN

Insulin plays a major role in allowing the body's cells to take in proteins, fatty acids, and glucose. Insulin is like a key that opens a door to the body's cells, so the nutrients needed by the cells can get inside.

the body's fat cells), but nearly 100 percent of the carbohydrate you eat is broken down into glucose. Chewing and swallowing begin the digestive process of breaking down starches and larger sugar molecules into glucose. The enzymes in your mouth and your intestines complete the breakdown. The glucose is then absorbed into the bloodstream and travels throughout the body. That's when the pancreas plays a vital role.

The pancreas is a fist-size organ just behind your stomach. One of its jobs is to make enzymes for food digestion. But, the pancreas also plays another important role. It contains small groups of cells, the islets of Langerhans, that make hormones, which are released into your bloodstream. Some 80 percent of these islet cells are called "beta" cells that make two hormones: amylin and insulin. Amylin plays a secondary role in regulating appetite and the rate of digestion. Insulin plays a major role in allowing the body's cells to take in proteins, fatty acids, and glucose. Insulin is like a key that opens a door to the body's cells, so the nutrients needed by the cells can get inside. When a person who does not have diabetes eats any food, their blood glucose level rises. The beta cells detect this rise and release more insulin. The insulin goes to the liver, telling the liver to make less glucose. It also helps the liver, muscle, and fat cells to take up more glucose. This allows nutrients from the recently eaten food to enter and "feed" the body's cells, it keeps blood glucose from rising too high even after eating, and it allows the glucose level to return to a normal, healthy range quickly. When we go many hours without eating, such as between meals or during sleep, the insulin levels fall, causing the liver to make more glucose to provide energy

for the brain, heart, lungs, etc., until the next meal.

In a person with diabetes, this process doesn't work properly. Either the beta cells have lost the ability to produce insulin or the insulin does not do its job as well as it should. As a result, the amount of glucose in the blood rises and the body's cells become deprived of the fuel they need.

DIFFERENT TYPES OF DIABETES

There are three major types of diabetes: type 1 diabetes, type 2 diabetes, and gestational diabetes. Each type requires a different type of treatment.

TYPE 1 DIABETES

This type affects about 5 percent of all people with diabetes. It is sometimes referred to as juvenile diabetes, because there is a higher rate of diagnosis in children, but people of any age can develop type 1 diabetes. It may also be called insulin-dependent diabetes, because those with type 1 diabetes require insulin (via injections or an insulin pump) to not only control their blood glucose, but to stay alive.

TYPE 2 DIABETES

Type 2 diabetes is the most common form of diabetes. It is estimated that up to 90 percent of the people who have diabetes have type 2. The cause appears to be resistance to insulin's action compounded by a deficiency of insulin secretion.

People with type 2 diabetes are usually over age 35, are overweight, and have a family history of type 2 diabetes. Type 2 diabetes actually begins years before diagnosis, as an increasing resistance to insulin. This increasing resistance is the result of genetics, weight gain (especially abdominal fat), decreased activity, and aging. The major site of insulin resistance is the muscle tissue, which normally burns up the majority of the glucose in the bloodstream. When insulin has a difficult time "opening doors" on the body's cells, the pancreas tries to compensate by making more and more insulin. For some people, the pancreas is eventually unable to keep up with the increased workload. Blood glucose levels rise above normal after meals, and fasting glucose levels begin to remain above normal, too. Ironically, very high glucose levels can damage the beta cells, a condition called glucose toxicity. This further accelerates the breakdown of the pancreas' ability to control blood sugar levels. When glucose rises high enough to produce symptoms (excessive thirst, frequent urination, wounds that don't heal, for example), or when a complication such as a heart attack, stroke, visual disturbance, infection, numbness, or serious gum disease is treated, the diagnosis of type 2 diabetes is often made.

GESTATIONAL DIABETES

Gestational diabetes is diagnosed for the first time during pregnancy. It occurs in about 3 percent of all pregnancies. Gestational diabetes is diagnosed using a 3-hour glucose tolerance test. If any two of the glucose readings during the test exceed the upper limits of normal, the diagnosis is made. Rarely are the glucose levels high enough to harm the mother. The problem is the mother's blood. Extra glucose flows to the developing baby, which then produces extra insulin. This, in turn, causes the baby to grow too quickly, resulting in a difficult labor and delivery.

Throughout the pregnancy, the mother's insulin resistance and glucose levels increase, right up to delivery. In 97 percent of cases, the mother's glucose levels promptly return to normal after delivery. Many women with gestational diabetes can control their glucose levels during pregnancy through diet and

TYPE 1 DIABETES

Affects about 5 percent of all people with diabetes. May also be called insulin-dependent diabetes, due to insulin (via injections or an insulin pump) being required to not only control blood glucose, but to stay alive.

TYPE 2 DIABETES

Most common form of diabetes. The cause appears to be resistance to insulin's action compounded by a deficiency of insulin secretion.

GESTATIONAL

Diagnosed for the first time during pregnancy. It occurs in about 3 percent of all pregnancies. Women who have had gestational diabetes have a significantly greater chance of developing diabetes later in life.

exercise. Some, however, require insulin to keep glucose levels within a healthy range for the fetus.

Women who have had gestational diabetes have a significantly greater chance of developing diabetes later in life. Studies have shown that weight control and increased physical activity reduce the risk of future diabetes by as much as 50 percent.

YOUR DIABETES TOOL KIT

A diagnosis of diabetes can be disheartening, but there is plenty of good news. These days, you have many diabetes tools to help you keep your blood sugar under tight control and ward off the frightening complications. You simply need to understand how to apply them to your best advantage and to commit yourself to using them faithfully.

MONITORING YOUR GLUCOSE

Blood glucose monitoring is a vital part of the diabetes management process, and frequent self-monitoring is a key to successful care. By checking your glucose, you get a precise measurement of what your blood glucose level is so you can adjust your food, medication, or activity level accordingly. Knowing your glucose level also lets you see if your previous food, medication, or activity level brought your glucose to a desired range. It means for greater freedom to participate in any activities you choose and, therefore, far greater control over your life. The blood glucose values are like clues in a mystery novel. The more clues you have, the greater your ability to solve the mystery. Of course, the opposite can be true as well. The less you check, the fewer clues

you have and the more your diabetes remains a mystery to both you and your diabetes care team.

Checking your blood glucose on a regular basis allows you to know the ongoing status of your diabetes and will help you learn more about it and your body. Checking multiple times each day will give you even more information, helping you understand blood glucose patterns that occur when you eat certain foods and take specific medication doses, as well as how these are connected to your level of activity and stressors at home or work. Frequent checking also ensures that you can catch high or low levels quickly and respond to them with appropriate adjustments.

EATING FOR BETTER CONTROL

When you learned you had diabetes, you may have assumed you'd have to go on a special, restrictive diet. Perhaps you'd heard of people with diabetes who had to give up every food they enjoyed or who stopped going to certain events or restaurants because there was nothing they could eat there. Well, cheer up. You don't need to follow a "diabetic diet" anymore.

Your body needs adequate amounts of six essential nutrients to function normally. Three of these—water, vitamins, and minerals—provide no energy and do not affect blood glucose levels. The other three—carbohydrate, protein, and fat—provide your body with the energy it needs to work. This energy is measured in calories. Any food that contains calories can cause your blood glucose levels to rise. For your body to properly use these energy calories, it needs insulin. Whenever you eat, your food is digested and broken down or converted into your body's primary fuel source, glucose. While all energy nutrients are broken down into glucose, carbohydrates have a more direct effect on blood glucose levels. Protein and fat have a slower, more indirect effect on those levels. Understanding this can help you predict how food will affect your glucose levels.

GLUCOSE MONITORING IS A MUST

It gives a precise measurement of what your blood glucose level is so you can adjust your food, medication, or activity level accordingly.

Checking your levels multiple times each day will give you even more information, helping you understand blood glucose patterns that occur when you eat certain foods and take specific medication doses, as well as how these are connected to your level of activity and stressors at home or work.

To be successful in diabetes self-care, you need to make personal food choices that are compatible with your blood glucose goals and your tastes. Since carbohydrates have the greatest direct effect on glucose levels, determining the amount of carbohydrates that your body can manage well is a cornerstone in your glucose management. It's simple, really. But before you begin, you should take a close look at your perceptions, preconceptions, and habits regarding food and eating; they can make eating much more complicated than need be. Adjusting them can allow you to enjoy the freedom that simplicity brings—and allow you to enjoy eating while you control your diabetes.

To gain a better understanding of how to use food choices to control your blood sugar levels, you must pay attention to how individual foods act in your body.

The first step is for you to eat absolutely normally. Have the foods you usually eat, in the amounts you normally have, as frequently as you usually have them. Check food labels to determine which foods contain carbohydrate, then keep a running tally of the total grams of carbohydrate you eat throughout the entire day. Take detailed, honest notes.

Along with taking these notes, you need to test your blood glucose levels. Testing allows you to see how well your insulin level matches your carbohydrate intake. No matter its source, insulin works with the food you eat. If you eat too much food for the insulin that is available, your glucose level will be too high; if you eat too little, your glucose level will be too low.

It is important to know that any food has the ability to make blood sugar levels rise, but different types of food as well as different amounts will result in different blood sugar levels. You may find that overeating makes blood sugar levels increase rapidly and stay too high. Overeating may not allow insulin to do its job properly. If you listen to your body's hunger cues and respect the feeling of fullness, your blood glucose will rise more slowly and peak at a lower level. Insulin, in turn, will be able to do its job and keep blood sugars at a healthy level. This type of balanced eating helps control diabetes and helps you feel better.

Eating a variety of foods will also help ensure that you get the nutrients you need—not just the carbohydrate, protein, and fat but also the vitamins and minerals that are essential to good health.

DIETARY CONTROL

Your body needs adequate amounts of six essential nutrients to function normally: water, vitamins, minerals, carbohydrates, protein, and fat. The last three provide your body with the energy it needs to work. This energy is measured in calories. Any food that contains calories can cause your blood glucose levels to rise. For your body to properly use these energy calories, it needs insulin. To be successful in diabetes self-care, you need to make personal food choices that are compatible with your blood glucose goals and your tastes.

STAYING ACTIVE

Activity is one of the three cornerstones in the treatment of diabetes, along with food and medication. Moving toward a more physically active life is generally inexpensive, convenient, and easy and usually produces great rewards in terms of blood glucose control (due to improved insulin sensitivity) and a general feeling of well-being.

Being active needs to be fun. Otherwise, you're much less likely to stick with an active lifestyle. So, choose your activities accordingly, then go out and play at least a little every day.

USING MEDICATIONS TO TREAT DIABETES

For many people who have type 2 diabetes, using food and activity to control blood glucose is not enough. For them, diabetes medications can be lifesavers—helping to lower blood glucose levels and stave off diabetes complications.

People with type 1 diabetes make very little, if any, insulin, so they are dependent on insulin injections. Insulin injections have become extremely safe and simple, and virtually pain-free. And, they remain the most natural and effective way to treat high blood sugar in these individuals.

On the other hand, individuals with type 2 diabetes may depend on pills to help lower blood glucose levels. But there are usually multiple problems that need to be addressed, and one pill just can't do it all. Problems include insulin resistance by the body's cells, oversecretion of glucose by the liver, insufficient insulin production by the pancreas, and alternated rates of food digestion. Sometimes a combination of medications is much more effective at lowering glucose levels than is a single medicine.

WEIGHING THE BENEFITS

You may realize (or your doctor has told you) that being overweight—especially carrying too much fat in your abdominal area—hampers diabetes control. For people with diabetes, the best path to weight loss is the same one that leads to getting well and staying well. There's no denying weight loss is beneficial for people with type 2 diabetes who are overweight. Even a weight loss of just 5 to 10 percent of your total body weight can bring impressive

BASICALLY, CHANGES THAT WILL HELP IMPROVE YOUR GLUCOSE CONTROL INCLUDE:

- **FILLING UP ON FIBER.** Foods high in fiber can help you feel fuller longer with fewer calories and without increasing blood sugar.

- **THINK SMALL.** Choose smaller, more reasonable portions on a smaller plate, and eat more slowly so you'll know it when your stomach is full.

- **CHECK THIRST.** Most people confuse feelings of thirst for hunger. Try reaching for a low-calorie beverage or water first before eating.

- **MAKE TRADES.** Choose foods that are lower in fat and light in calories instead of a higher calorie/fat dense food.

- **ADD MORE ACTIVITY.** The more you move, the more you'll lose.

improvements to your health. Studies show that when a person who has recently been diagnosed with diabetes loses weight, blood glucose levels drop, blood pressure improves, and cholesterol levels return to a healthier range. Medications may be decreased or even stopped altogether.

TAKING COMMAND OF YOUR CARE

The right approach to diabetes treatment puts YOU in charge. Not your doctor. Not your spouse. YOU. You become the boss of your diabetes team, choosing the staff that best serves your needs, tracking your progress, and keeping your eyes on the ultimate goal—your health and well-being.

YOUR DIABETES TEAM

Surround yourself with knowledgeable, trustworthy, and expert advisors—your diabetes care team—who can help your get the information, advice, treatments, and support you need to manage your diabetes effectively. This team should include your doctor (possibly an endocrinologist who typically has the most experience and skill in diabetes care) and a registered dietitian nutritionist (RDN) who may also be certified as a diabetes educator (CDE) to teach people with diabetes how to manage the disease. Also onboard should be a pharmacist, dentist, mental-health professional, eye doctor, podiatrist, and cardiologist, as needed.

Your team will help you choose what, how much, and when to eat; help you become more physically active; assist with your medications; check your blood glucose; and teach you all they can about diabetes.

YOU'RE ON YOUR WAY

Once you feel comfortable with your meal and activity plan, checking your blood sugar, and managing your medication, you'll be able to enjoy the great taste of food without worries. Use the following recipes to get started on the path to a healthier lifestyle.

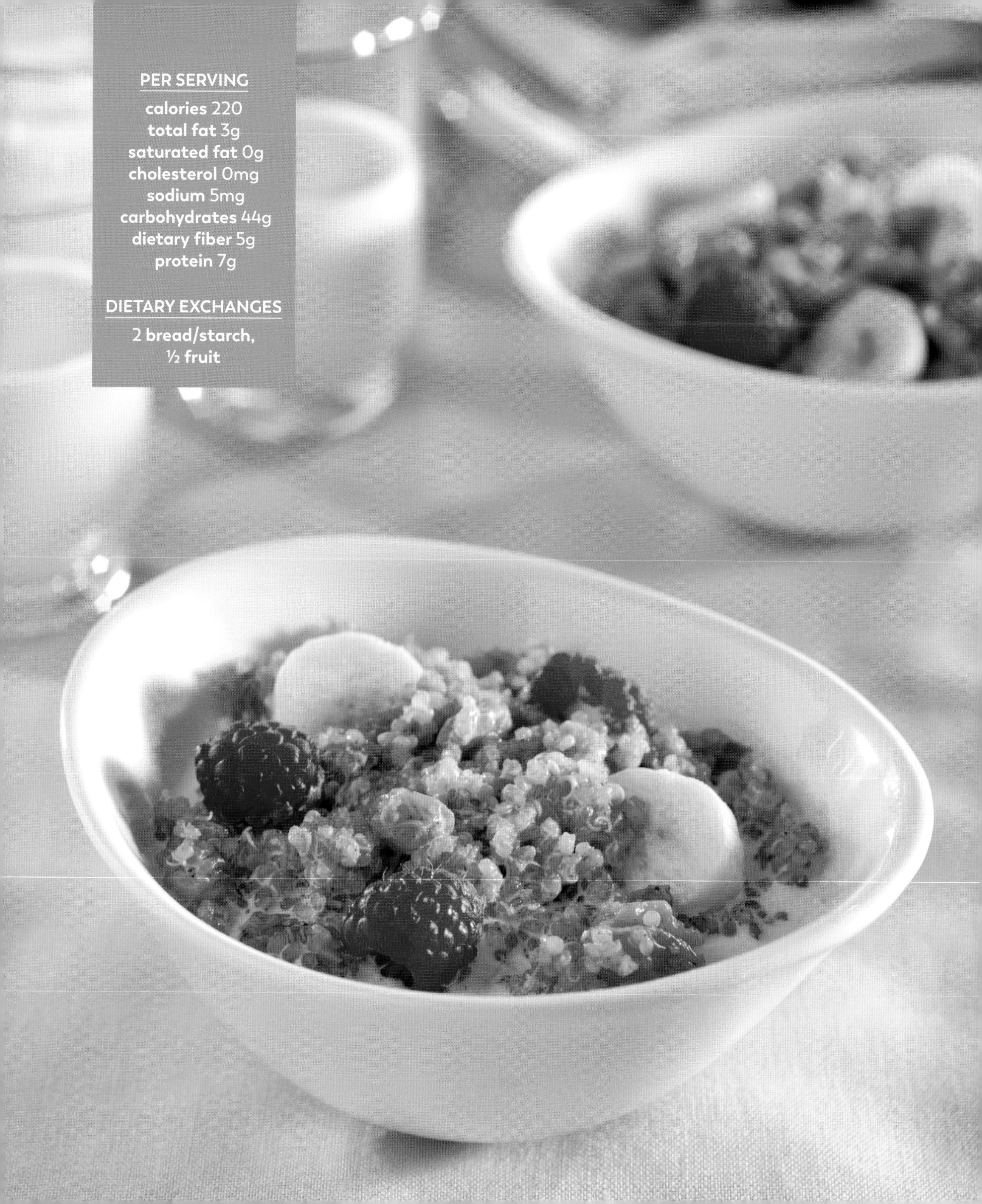

PER SERVING

calories 220
total fat 3g
saturated fat 0g
cholesterol 0mg
sodium 5mg
carbohydrates 44g
dietary fiber 5g
protein 7g

DIETARY EXCHANGES

2 **bread/starch,**
½ **fruit**

busy-day breakfasts

Breakfast Quinoa

Makes 2 servings

- ½ cup uncooked quinoa
- 1 cup water
- 1 tablespoon packed brown sugar
- 2 teaspoons sugar-free maple syrup
- ½ teaspoon ground cinnamon
- ¼ cup golden raisins (optional)
  Milk (optional)
- ¼ cup fresh raspberries
- ½ banana, sliced

1. Place quinoa in fine-mesh strainer; rinse well under cold running water. Transfer to small saucepan.

2. Stir in 1 cup water, brown sugar, maple syrup and cinnamon; bring to a boil over high heat. Reduce heat to low; cover and simmer 10 to 15 minutes or until quinoa is tender and water is absorbed. Add raisins, if desired, during last 5 minutes of cooking. Serve with milk, if desired; top with raspberries and bananas.

Sweet & Savory Breakfast Muffins

Makes 12 muffins

1¼ cups original pancake and baking mix

1 cup fat-free (skim) milk

3 egg whites

¼ cup sugar-free maple syrup

4 small fully cooked turkey breakfast sausage links, diced

1 cup fresh blueberries

1. Preheat oven to 375°F. Spray 12 standard (2½-inch) muffin cups with nonstick cooking spray.

2. Stir pancake mix, milk, egg whites and maple syrup in large bowl until smooth and well blended. Fold in sausage and blueberries. Pour evenly into prepared muffin cups.

3. Bake 18 to 20 minutes or until toothpick inserted into centers comes out clean. Serve warm.

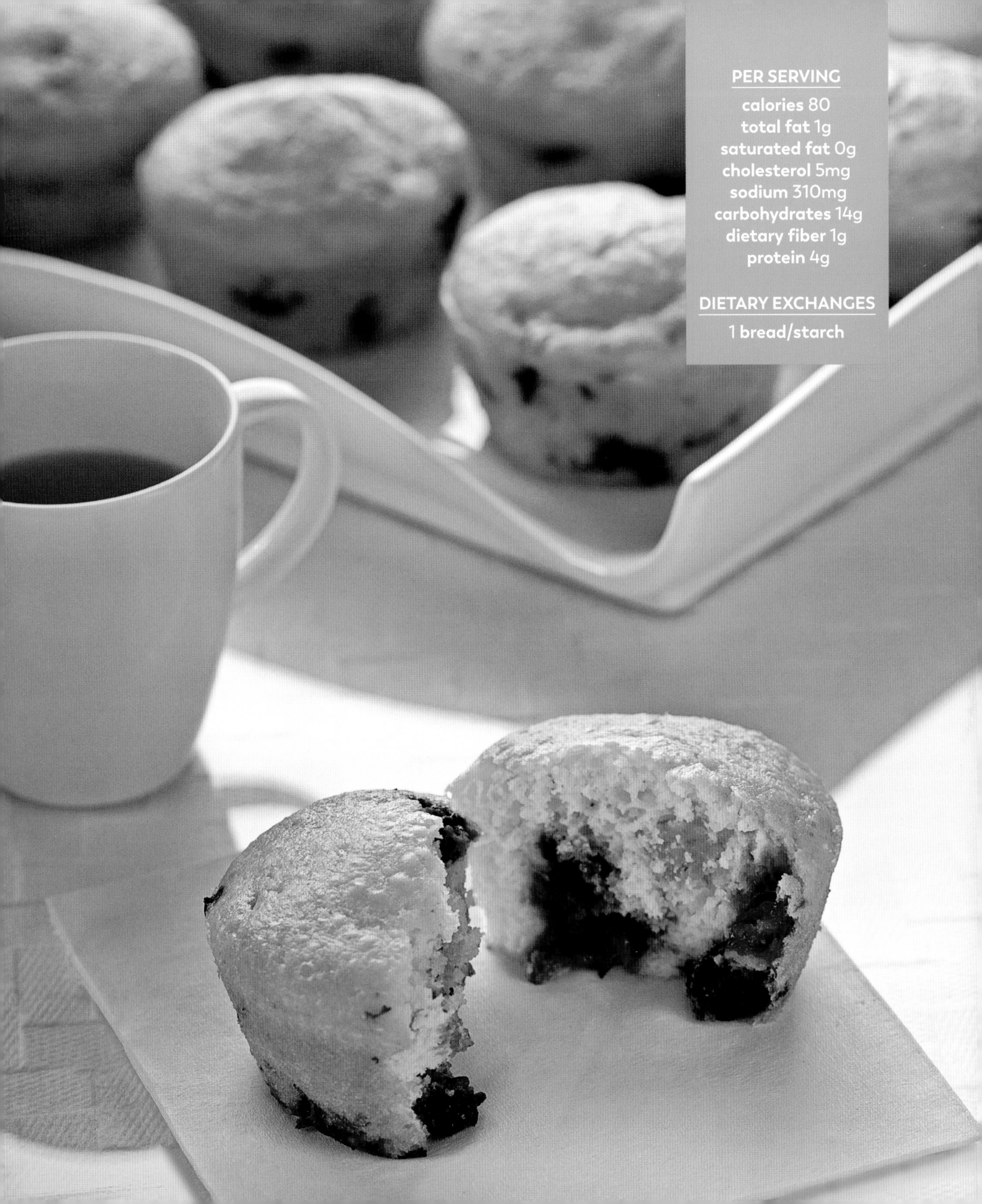

PER SERVING

calories 80
total fat 1g
saturated fat 0g
cholesterol 5mg
sodium 310mg
carbohydrates 14g
dietary fiber 1g
protein 4g

DIETARY EXCHANGES

1 bread/starch

Harvest Apple Oatmug

Makes 1 serving

1 cup water

½ cup old-fashioned oats

½ cup chopped Granny Smith apple

2 tablespoons raisins

1 teaspoon packed brown sugar

¼ teaspoon ground cinnamon

⅛ teaspoon salt

Microwave Directions

1. Combine water, oats, apple, raisins, brown sugar, cinnamon and salt in large microwavable mug; mix well.

2. Microwave on HIGH 1½ minutes; stir. Microwave on HIGH 1 minute or until thickened and liquid is absorbed. Let stand 1 to 2 minutes before serving.

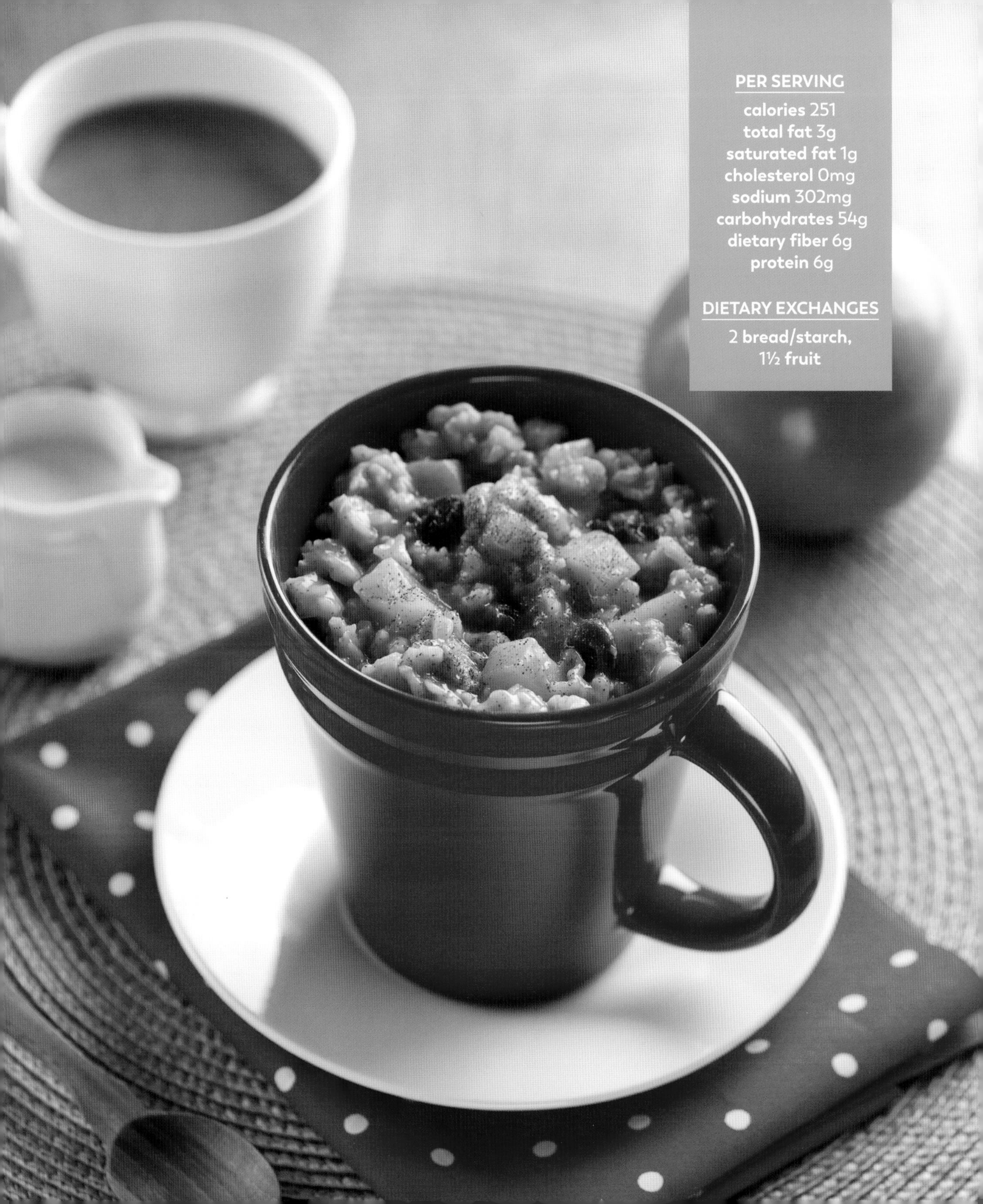

PER SERVING

calories 251
total fat 3g
saturated fat 1g
cholesterol 0mg
sodium 302mg
carbohydrates 54g
dietary fiber 6g
protein 6g

DIETARY EXCHANGES

2 **bread/starch,**
1½ **fruit**

Zucchini Bread Pancakes

Makes 3 servings (2 pancakes per serving)

1 medium zucchini, grated

¼ cup vanilla nonfat yogurt

1 egg

2 tablespoons fat-free (skim) milk

1 tablespoon vegetable oil

½ cup whole wheat flour

2 tablespoons packed brown sugar

1 teaspoon grated lemon peel, plus additional for garnish

1 teaspoon baking soda

½ teaspoon ground cinnamon

⅛ teaspoon ground nutmeg

Sugar-free maple syrup (optional)

1. Combine zucchini, yogurt, egg, milk and oil in large bowl; mix well. Add flour, brown sugar, 1 teaspoon lemon peel, baking soda, cinnamon and nutmeg; stir just until combined.

2. Heat large nonstick griddle or skillet over medium-low heat. Pour ¼ cupfuls of batter 2 inches apart onto griddle. Cook 3 minutes or until lightly browned and edges begin to bubble. Turn over; cook 3 minutes or until lightly browned. Repeat with remaining batter.

3. Serve with maple syrup, if desired. Garnish with additional lemon peel.

PER SERVING
calories 198
total fat 7g
saturated fat 1g
cholesterol 63mg
sodium 468mg
carbohydrates 29g
dietary fiber 3g
protein 7g

DIETARY EXCHANGES
2 bread/starch,
½ vegetable

Breakfast Pizza Margherita

Makes 6 servings

- 1 (12-inch) prepared pizza crust
- 3 slices 95% fat-free turkey bacon
- 2 cups cholesterol-free egg substitute
- ½ cup fat-free (skim) milk
- 1½ tablespoons chopped fresh basil, divided
- ⅛ teaspoon black pepper
- 2 plum tomatoes, thinly sliced
- ½ cup (2 ounces) shredded reduced-fat mozzarella cheese
- ¼ cup (1 ounce) shredded reduced-fat Cheddar cheese

1. Preheat oven to 450°F. Place pizza crust on 12-inch pizza pan. Bake 6 to 8 minutes or until heated through.

2. Meanwhile, coat large skillet with nonstick cooking spray. Cook bacon over medium-high heat until crisp. Remove from skillet to paper towels; cool. Crumble bacon.

3. Combine egg substitute, milk, ½ tablespoon basil and pepper in medium bowl. Coat same skillet with cooking spray. Add egg substitute mixture. Cook over medium heat until mixture begins to set around edges. Gently stir eggs, allowing uncooked portions to flow underneath. Repeat stirring of egg mixture every 1 to 2 minutes or until eggs are just set. Remove from heat.

4. Arrange tomato slices on warmed pizza crust. Spoon scrambled eggs over tomatoes. Sprinkle with bacon. Top with cheeses. Bake 1 minute or until cheeses are melted. Sprinkle with remaining 1 tablespoon basil. Cut into six wedges. Serve immediately.

PER SERVING
calories 311
total fat 9g
saturated fat 2g
cholesterol 11mg
sodium 675mg
carbohydrates 35g
dietary fiber 2g
protein 21g

DIETARY EXCHANGES
2 bread/starch,
2 meat, ½ vegetable,
1½ fat

Fruited Granola

Makes 20 servings (about ½ cup per serving)

3 cups quick-cooking oats

1 cup sliced almonds

1 cup honey

½ cup wheat germ or honey wheat germ

3 tablespoons butter or margarine, melted

1 teaspoon ground cinnamon

3 cups whole grain cereal flakes

½ cup dried blueberries or golden raisins

½ cup dried cranberries or cherries

½ cup dried banana chips or chopped pitted dates

1. Preheat oven to 325°F.

2. Spread oats and almonds in single layer in 13×9-inch baking pan. Bake 15 minutes or until lightly toasted, stirring frequently.

3. Combine honey, wheat germ, butter and cinnamon in large bowl until well blended. Add oats and almonds; toss to coat completely. Spread mixture in single layer in baking pan. Bake 20 minutes or until golden brown. Cool completely in pan on wire rack. Break mixture into chunks.

4. Combine oat chunks, cereal, blueberries, cranberries and banana chips in large bowl. Store in airtight container at room temperature up to 2 weeks.

Tip: Prepare this granola on the weekend and you'll have a scrumptious snack or breakfast treat on hand for the rest of the week!

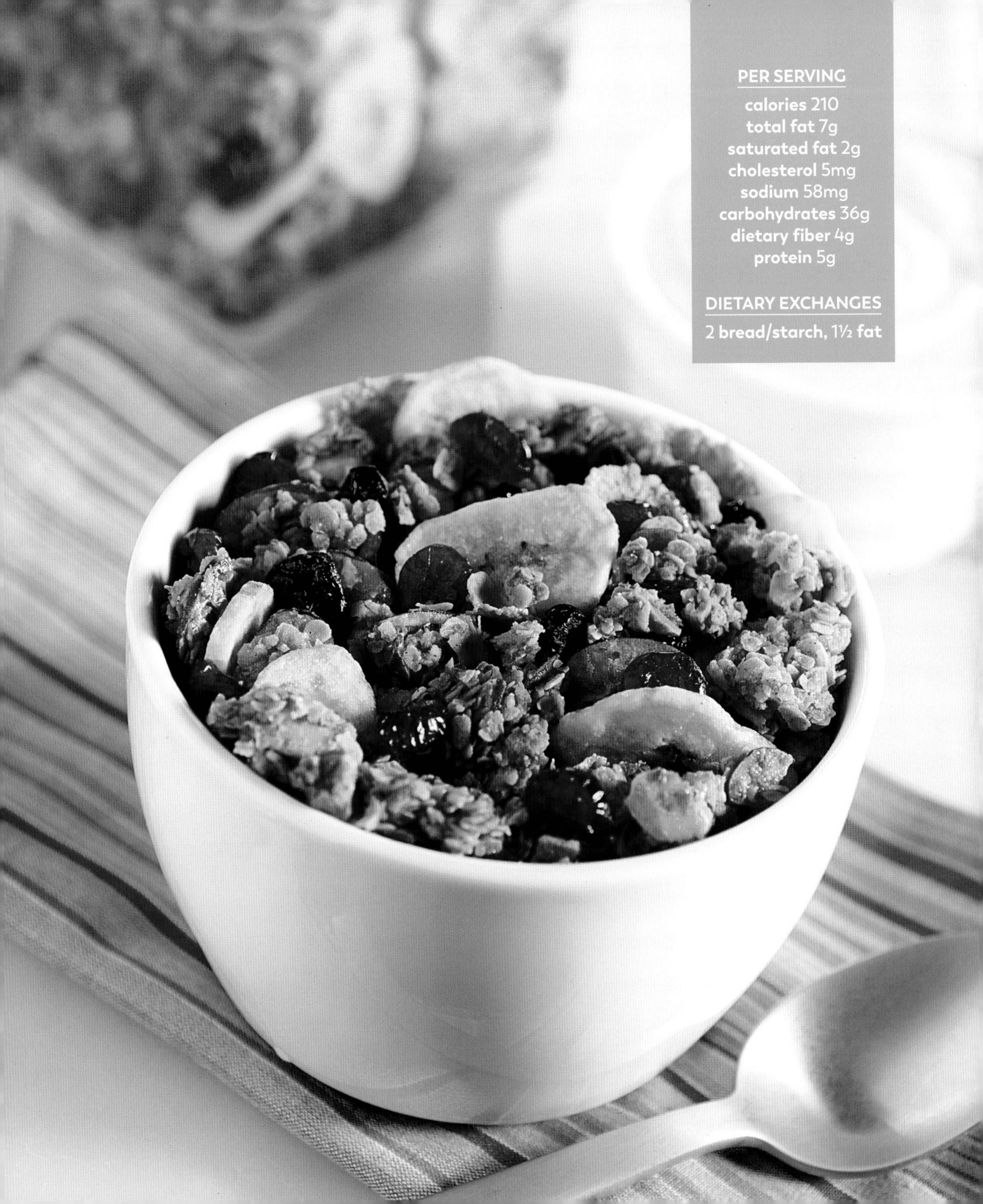

PER SERVING

calories 210
total fat 7g
saturated fat 2g
cholesterol 5mg
sodium 58mg
carbohydrates 36g
dietary fiber 4g
protein 5g

DIETARY EXCHANGES

2 bread/starch, 1½ fat

Baked Ginger Pear Oatmeal

Makes 2 servings

1   cup old-fashioned oats

¾   cup fat-free (skim) milk

1   egg white

2   tablespoons packed brown
     sugar, divided

1½ teaspoons grated fresh ginger
     or ¾ teaspoon ground ginger

½   ripe pear, diced

1. Preheat oven to 350°F. Spray two (6-ounce) ramekins with nonstick cooking spray.

2. Combine oats, milk, egg white, 1 tablespoon brown sugar and ginger in medium bowl; mix well. Pour evenly into ramekins. Top with pear; sprinkle with remaining 1 tablespoon brown sugar.

3. Bake 15 minutes. Serve warm.

PER SERVING
calories 268
total fat 3g
saturated fat 1g
cholesterol 2mg
sodium 70mg
carbohydrates 52g
dietary fiber 5g
protein 10g

DIETARY EXCHANGES
3½ **bread/starch**

German Apple Pancake

Makes 6 servings

- 1 tablespoon butter
- 1 large *or* 2 small apples, peeled and thinly sliced (about 1½ cups)
- 1 tablespoon packed brown sugar
- 1½ teaspoons ground cinnamon, divided
- 2 eggs
- 2 egg whites
- 1 tablespoon granulated sugar
- 1 teaspoon vanilla
- ¼ teaspoon salt
- ½ cup all-purpose flour
- ½ cup milk
- Sugar-free maple syrup (optional)

1. Preheat oven to 425°F.

2. Melt butter in medium cast iron or ovenproof skillet* over medium heat. Add apples, brown sugar and ½ teaspoon cinnamon; cook and stir 5 minutes or until apples just begin to soften. Remove from heat. Arrange apple slices in single layer in skillet.

3. Whisk eggs, egg whites, granulated sugar, remaining 1 teaspoon cinnamon, vanilla and salt in medium bowl until well blended. Stir in flour and milk until smooth and well blended. Pour evenly over apples.

4. Bake 20 to 25 minutes or until puffed and golden brown. Serve with maple syrup, if desired.

To make skillet ovenproof, wrap handle in foil.

Note: Pancake will fall slightly after being removed from the oven.

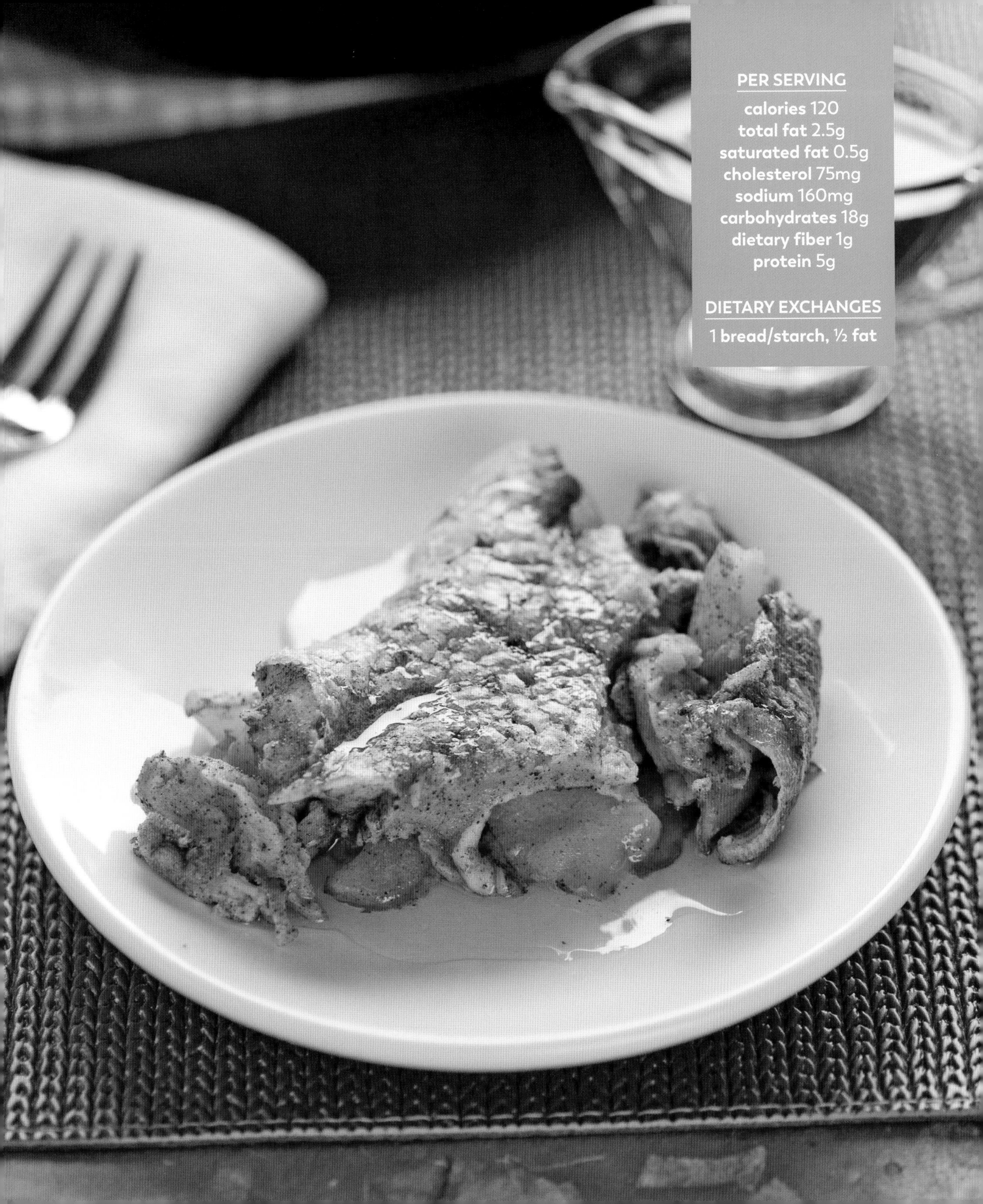

PER SERVING

calories 120
total fat 2.5g
saturated fat 0.5g
cholesterol 75mg
sodium 160mg
carbohydrates 18g
dietary fiber 1g
protein 5g

DIETARY EXCHANGES

1 bread/starch, ½ fat

Very Berry Yogurt Parfaits

Makes 4 servings

3 cups plain nonfat yogurt

2 tablespoons sugar-free berry preserves

1 packet sugar substitute*

½ teaspoon vanilla

2 cups sliced fresh strawberries

1 cup fresh blueberries

4 tablespoons sliced toasted almonds

This recipe was tested with sucralose-based sugar substitute.

1. Combine yogurt, preserves, sugar substitute and vanilla in medium bowl.

2. Layer ½ cup yogurt mixture, ¼ cup strawberries, ¼ cup blueberries and ¼ cup yogurt mixture in each of four dessert dishes. Top each parfait with remaining ¼ cup strawberries and 1 tablespoon almonds. Serve immediately.

Notes: These parfaits would also be delicious topped with low-fat granola. Or, try another flavor of preserves for a simple variation.

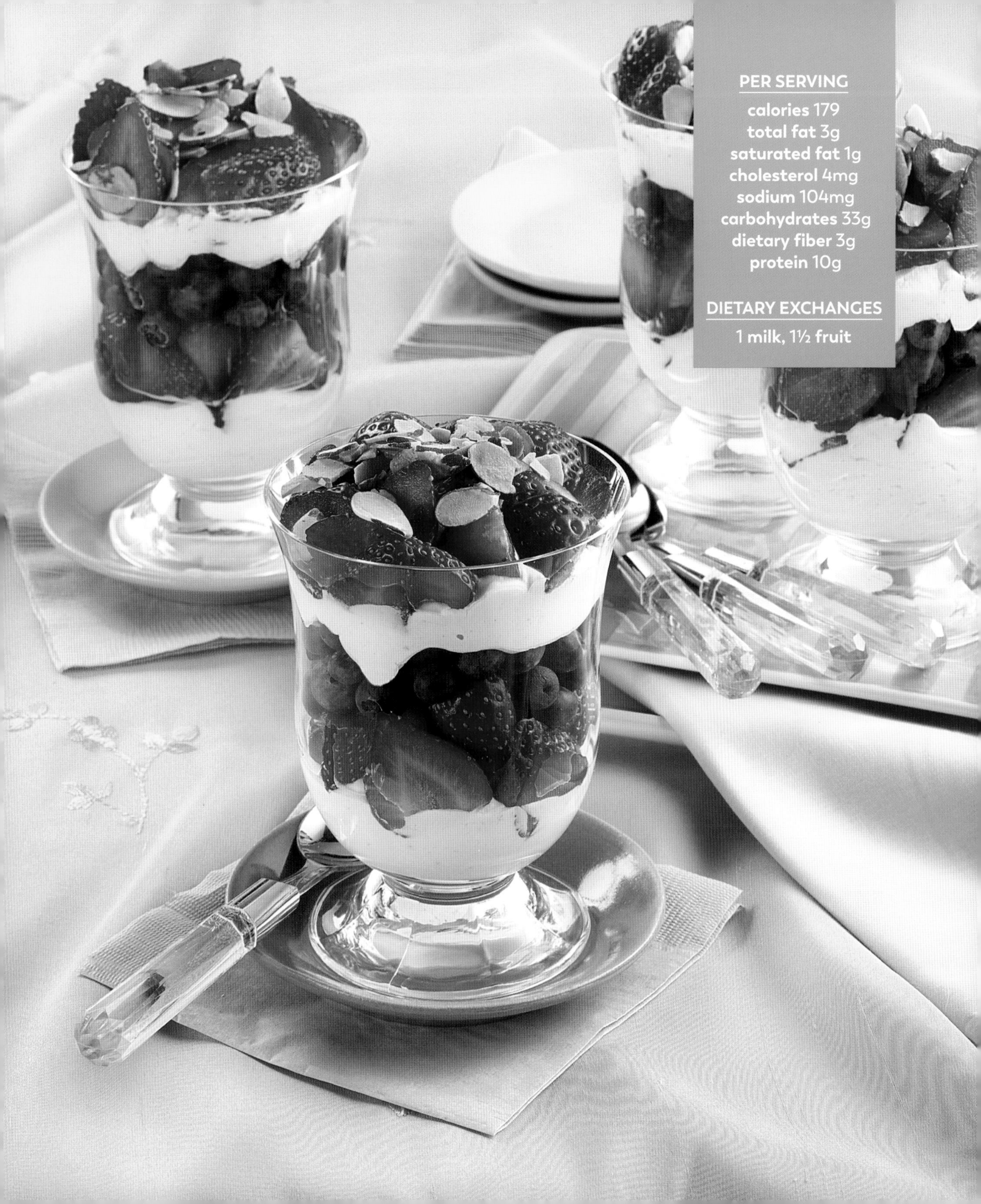

PER SERVING

calories 179
total fat 3g
saturated fat 1g
cholesterol 4mg
sodium 104mg
carbohydrates 33g
dietary fiber 3g
protein 10g

DIETARY EXCHANGES

1 milk, 1½ fruit

light *and* tasty lunches

Chicken Satay Salad

Makes 4 servings

¼ cup plus 2 tablespoons peanut sauce, divided

2 tablespoons lime juice

1 tablespoon unseasoned rice vinegar

3 teaspoons toasted sesame oil, divided

1 pound chicken tenders, cut in half lengthwise

4 cups chopped romaine lettuce

1 red bell pepper, thinly sliced

1 cup shredded carrots

1 cup sliced Persian cucumbers*

¼ cup chopped fresh cilantro

1 tablespoon peanuts, chopped

*Persian cucumbers are similar to English cucumbers; they have fewer seeds and contain less water than traditional cucumbers, which gives them a sweeter flavor and crunchier texture. These smaller cucumbers can be found in packages of six in the produce section of the supermarket.

1. Whisk ¼ cup peanut sauce, lime juice, vinegar and 1 teaspoon oil in large bowl until smooth and well blended. Set aside.

2. Heat remaining 2 teaspoons oil in large nonstick skillet over medium-high heat. Add chicken; cook and stir 4 minutes or until chicken is no longer pink. Remove from heat. Add remaining 2 tablespoons peanut sauce; gently toss to coat evenly.

3. Add lettuce, bell pepper, carrots and cucumbers to dressing in large bowl; toss to coat.

4. Divide salad evenly among four plates. Top with chicken, cilantro and peanuts.

Summer's Bounty Pasta with Broccoli Pesto

Makes 4 servings

2 cups broccoli florets

2 cups uncooked farfalle (bowtie pasta)

½ cup loosely packed fresh basil leaves

5 tablespoons shredded Parmesan-Romano cheese blend, divided

2 tablespoons chopped walnuts, toasted*

1½ tablespoons extra virgin olive oil

2 cloves garlic, crushed and divided

⅛ teaspoon salt

6 ounces medium cooked shrimp

¼ teaspoon black pepper

1 package (6 ounces) fresh baby spinach

1 cup halved grape tomatoes

To toast walnuts, spread in heavy skillet. Cook over medium heat 1 to 2 minutes or until nuts are lightly browned, stirring frequently.

1. Bring large saucepan of water to a boil. Add broccoli; cook 3 minutes or until tender. Remove to small bowl with slotted spoon; reserve water.

2. Cook pasta according to package directions using reserved water, omitting salt. Drain pasta; cover to keep warm.

3. Combine broccoli, basil, 3 tablespoons cheese, walnuts, oil, 1 clove garlic and salt in food processor or blender; process until smooth. Stir into pasta in saucepan; toss to coat. Cover to keep warm.

4. Spray large skillet with nonstick cooking spray; heat over medium heat. Add shrimp, remaining 1 clove garlic and pepper; cook and stir until heated through. Stir in spinach and tomatoes; cook until spinach is wilted and tomatoes begin to soften. Add to pasta; stir gently to combine.

5. Divide pasta mixture evenly among four serving bowls; top with remaining 2 tablespoons cheese.

Wild Mushroom Tofu Burgers

Makes 6 servings

3 teaspoons olive oil, divided

1 package (8 ounces) cremini mushrooms, roughly chopped

½ medium onion, roughly chopped

1 clove garlic, minced

7 ounces extra firm lite tofu, crumbled and frozen

1 cup old-fashioned oats

⅓ cup finely chopped walnuts

1 egg

½ teaspoon salt

½ teaspoon onion powder

¼ teaspoon dried thyme

6 light multi-grain English muffins, split and toasted

Lettuce, tomato and red onion slices (optional)

Cucumber spears (optional)

1. Heat 1 teaspoon oil in large nonstick skillet over medium heat. Add mushrooms, onion and garlic; cook and stir 10 minutes or until mushrooms have released most of their juices. Remove from heat; cool slightly.

2. Combine mushroom mixture, tofu, oats, walnuts, egg, salt, onion powder and thyme in food processor or blender; process until combined. (Some tofu pieces may remain). Shape mixture into six (⅓-cup) patties.

3. Heat 1 teaspoon oil in same skillet over medium-low heat. Working in batches, cook patties 5 minutes per side. Repeat with remaining oil and patties.

4. Serve burgers on English muffins with lettuce, tomato and red onion, if desired. Garnish with cucumber spears.

PER SERVING
calories 254
total fat 10g
saturated fat 1g
cholesterol 31mg
sodium 469mg
carbohydrates 37g
dietary fiber 9g
protein 13g

DIETARY EXCHANGES
2½ bread/starch,
1 meat, 1 fat

Quinoa Burrito Bowls

Makes 4 servings

- 1 cup uncooked quinoa
- 2 cups water
- 2 tablespoons fresh lime juice, divided
- ¼ cup light sour cream
- 2 teaspoons vegetable oil
- 1 small onion, diced
- 1 red bell pepper, diced
- 1 clove garlic, minced
- ½ cup canned black beans, rinsed and drained
- ½ cup thawed frozen corn
- Shredded lettuce
- Lime wedges (optional)

1. Place quinoa in fine-mesh strainer; rinse well under cold running water. Bring 2 cups water to a boil in small saucepan; stir in quinoa. Reduce heat to low; cover and simmer 10 to 15 minutes or until quinoa is tender and water is absorbed. Stir in 1 tablespoon lime juice. Cover and keep warm. Combine sour cream and remaining 1 tablespoon lime juice in small bowl; set aside.

2. Meanwhile, heat oil in large skillet over medium heat. Add onion and bell pepper; cook and stir 5 minutes or until softened. Add garlic; cook 1 minute. Add black beans and corn; cook 3 to 5 minutes or until heated through.

3. Divide quinoa among four serving bowls; top with black bean mixture, lettuce and sour cream mixture. Garnish with lime wedges.

PER SERVING
calories 258
total fat 7g
saturated fat 1g
cholesterol 4mg
sodium 136mg
carbohydrates 42g
dietary fiber 6g
protein 9g

DIETARY EXCHANGES
3 bread/starch, 1 fat

Roasted Eggplant Panini

Makes 4 sandwiches

1 medium eggplant (about 1¼ pounds)

1 cup (4 ounces) shredded reduced-fat mozzarella cheese

1 tablespoon chopped fresh basil

1 tablespoon fresh lemon juice

⅛ teaspoon salt

8 slices (1 ounce each) whole grain Italian bread

1. Preheat oven to 400°F. Line baking sheet with parchment paper; spray with nonstick cooking spray. Slice eggplant in half lengthwise. Place cut sides down on prepared baking sheet. Roast 45 minutes. Let stand 15 minutes or until cool enough to handle.

2. Meanwhile, combine cheese, basil, lemon juice and salt in small bowl; set aside.

3. Cut each eggplant piece in half. Remove pulp; discard skin. Place one fourth of eggplant on each of 4 bread slices, pressing gently into bread. Top evenly with cheese mixture. Top with remaining bread slices. Spray sandwiches with cooking spray.

4. Heat large nonstick grill pan or skillet over medium heat. Cook sandwiches 3 to 4 minutes per side, pressing down with spatula until cheese is melted and bread is toasted. (Cover pan during last minute of cooking to melt cheese, if desired.) Serve immediately.

PER SERVING

calories 310
total fat 7g
saturated fat 2g
cholesterol 10mg
sodium 275mg
carbohydrates 50g
dietary fiber 9g
protein 19g

DIETARY EXCHANGES

3 bread/starch,
2 meat

Salmon Caesar Salad

Makes 1 serving

1 skinless salmon fillet (4 ounces)

3 cups chopped romaine lettuce

1 tablespoon light creamy Caesar salad dressing

6 fat-free croutons

1 teaspoon grated Parmesan cheese

1. Spray small skillet with nonstick cooking spray; heat over medium heat. Add salmon; cook 4 minutes per side or until salmon flakes easily when tested with fork. When cool enough to handle, cut into bite-size pieces.

2. Meanwhile, combine lettuce and dressing in medium bowl; toss to coat evenly.

3. Arrange lettuce on plate. Top with salmon, croutons and cheese.

PER SERVING
calories 263
total fat 11g
saturated fat 2g
cholesterol 63mg
sodium 344mg
carbohydrates 12g
dietary fiber 3g
protein 26g

DIETARY EXCHANGES
½ bread/starch,
3 meat, 1 vegetable,
1 fat

Turkey & Veggie Roll-Ups

Makes 2 servings

2 tablespoons hummus, any flavor

1 (8-inch) whole wheat tortilla

¼ cup sliced baby spinach

2 slices oven-roasted turkey breast (about 1 ounce)

¼ cup thinly sliced English cucumber

1 slice (1 ounce) reduced-fat Swiss cheese

¼ cup thinly sliced carrot

Spread hummus on tortilla to within 1 inch of edge. Layer with spinach, turkey, cucumber, cheese and carrots. Roll up tortilla and filling; cut into four pieces.

PER SERVING
calories 140
total fat 4g
saturated fat 1g
cholesterol 16mg
sodium 292mg
carbohydrates 14g
dietary fiber 2g
protein 11g

DIETARY EXCHANGES
1 bread/starch,
1 meat

Mandarin Chicken Salad

Makes 4 servings

3½ ounces thin rice noodles (rice vermicelli)

1 can (6 ounces) mandarin orange segments, chilled

⅓ cup honey

2 tablespoons rice wine vinegar

2 tablespoons reduced-sodium soy sauce

1 can (8 ounces) sliced water chestnuts, drained

4 cups shredded napa cabbage

1 cup shredded red cabbage

½ cup sliced radishes

4 thin slices red onion, cut in half and separated

3 boneless skinless chicken breasts (about 12 ounces), cooked and cut into strips

1. Place rice noodles in large bowl. Cover with hot water; soak 20 minutes or until soft. Drain.

2. Drain mandarin orange segments, reserving ⅓ cup liquid. Whisk reserved liquid, honey, vinegar and soy sauce in medium bowl. Add water chestnuts.

3. Divide noodles, cabbages, radishes and onion evenly among four serving plates. Top with chicken and orange segments. Remove water chestnuts from dressing and arrange on salads. Serve with remaining dressing.

PER SERVING
calories 258
total fat 2g
saturated fat 1g
cholesterol 34mg
sodium 318mg
carbohydrates 46g
dietary fiber 2g
protein 16g

DIETARY EXCHANGES
1 bread/starch,
2 meat, 2 vegetable,
½ fruit

Mediterranean Tuna Salad

Makes 4 servings

- 1 cup diced tomato
- 1 tablespoon olive oil
- 1 tablespoon lemon juice
- 2 teaspoons Dijon mustard
- 1 clove garlic, minced
- ¼ teaspoon salt
- ¼ teaspoon dried basil
- 2 cans (5 ounces each) solid white tuna packed in water, drained and flaked
- ½ cup diced celery
- ⅓ cup chopped fresh basil
- Red leaf lettuce leaves
- ½ pound steamed green beans
- 1 medium red bell pepper, seeded and cut into strips
- 8 cherry tomatoes, halved

1. Combine diced tomato, oil, lemon juice, mustard, garlic, salt and dried basil in large bowl; let stand 5 minutes. Stir in tuna, celery and fresh basil. Refrigerate, covered, 1 to 2 hours to allow flavors to blend, stirring once.

2. Line serving platter with lettuce leaves. Mound tuna salad in center; serve with green beans, bell pepper and cherry tomatoes.

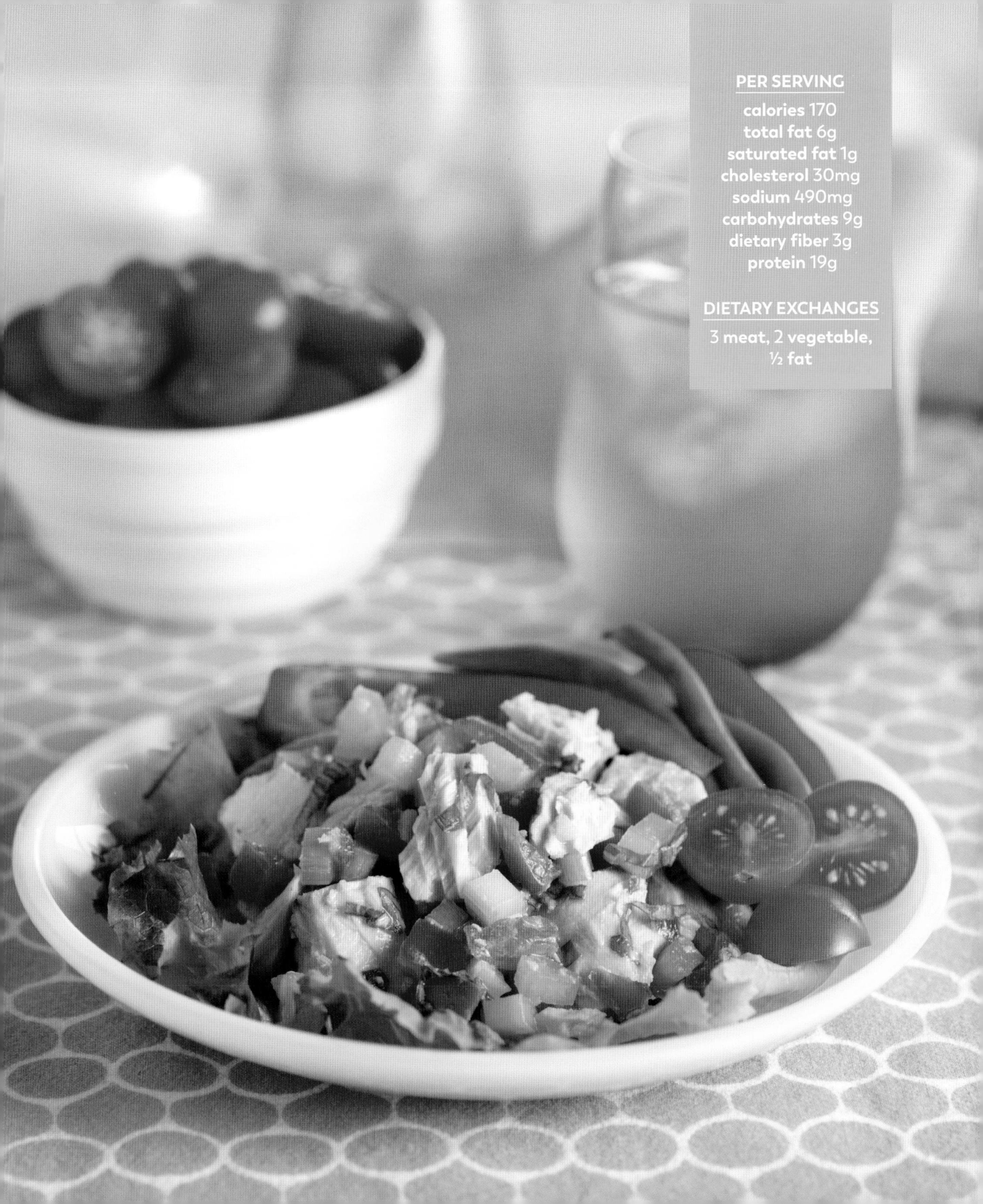

PER SERVING

calories 170
total fat 6g
saturated fat 1g
cholesterol 30mg
sodium 490mg
carbohydrates 9g
dietary fiber 3g
protein 19g

DIETARY EXCHANGES

3 **meat**, 2 **vegetable**, ½ **fat**

Pesto Tuna Melts

Makes 2 servings

- 1 can (5 ounces) tuna in water, drained and flaked
- 1 tablespoon plain nonfat Greek yogurt
- 1 tablespoon pesto sauce
- 1 teaspoon lemon juice
- ⅛ teaspoon black pepper
- 2 light multi-grain English muffins, split
- 4 tomato slices
- 6 teaspoons shredded reduced-fat mozzarella cheese

1. Preheat oven to 350°F.

2. Combine tuna, yogurt, pesto, lemon juice and pepper in small bowl; gently mix.

3. Divide tuna mixture evenly among English muffin halves. Top each half with 1 tomato slice and 1½ teaspoons cheese.

4. Bake 8 to 10 minutes or until cheese is melted.

PER SERVING
calories 270
total fat 6g
saturated fat 1g
cholesterol 30mg
sodium 580mg
carbohydrates 32g
dietary fiber 1g
protein 21g

DIETARY EXCHANGES
2 bread/starch,
2 meat, 1 fat

Vegetarian Paella

Makes 6 servings

- 2 teaspoons canola oil
- 1 cup chopped onion
- 2 cloves garlic, minced
- 1 cup uncooked brown rice
- 2¼ cups vegetable broth
- 1 can (about 14 ounces) no-salt-added stewed tomatoes
- 1 small zucchini, halved lengthwise and sliced to ½-inch thickness (about 1¼ cups)
- 1 cup chopped red bell pepper
- 2 teaspoons Italian seasoning
- ½ teaspoon ground turmeric
- ⅛ teaspoon ground red pepper
- 1 can (14 ounces) quartered artichoke hearts, drained
- ½ cup frozen baby peas
- ¾ teaspoon salt (optional)

Slow Cooker Directions

1. Heat oil in small nonstick skillet over medium-high heat. Add onion; cook and stir 6 to 7 minutes or until tender. Stir in garlic. Transfer to slow cooker. Stir in rice.

2. Add broth, tomatoes, zucchini, bell pepper, Italian seasoning, turmeric and ground red pepper; mix well. Cover; cook on LOW 4 hours or on HIGH 2 hours or until liquid is absorbed.

3. Stir in artichokes, peas and salt, if desired. Cover; cook on LOW 5 to 10 minutes or until vegetables are tender.

PER SERVING

calories 241
total fat 7g
saturated fat 1g
cholesterol 0mg
sodium 470mg
carbohydrates 43g
dietary fiber 7g
protein 5g

DIETARY EXCHANGES
3 bread/starch, 1 fat

Lentil Burgers

Makes 4 servings

- 1 can (about 14 ounces) vegetable broth
- 1 cup dried lentils, rinsed and sorted
- 1 small carrot, grated
- ¼ cup coarsely chopped mushrooms
- 1 egg
- ¼ cup plain dry bread crumbs
- 3 tablespoons finely chopped onion
- 2 to 4 cloves garlic, minced
- 1 teaspoon dried thyme
- ¼ cup plain fat-free yogurt
- ¼ cup chopped seeded cucumber
- ½ teaspoon dried mint
- ¼ teaspoon dried dill weed
- ¼ teaspoon black pepper
- ⅛ teaspoon salt
- Dash hot pepper sauce (optional)
- Kaiser rolls (optional)

1. Bring broth to a boil in medium saucepan over high heat. Stir in lentils; reduce heat to low. Simmer, covered, about 30 minutes or until lentils are tender and liquid is absorbed. Cool to room temperature.

2. Place lentils, carrot and mushrooms in food processor or blender; process until finely chopped but not smooth. (Some whole lentils should still be visible.) Stir in egg, bread crumbs, onion, garlic and thyme. Refrigerate, covered, 2 to 3 hours.

3. Shape lentil mixture into four (½-inch-thick) patties. Spray large skillet with nonstick cooking spray; heat over medium heat. Cook patties over medium-low heat about 10 minutes or until browned on both sides.

4. Meanwhile, for sauce, combine yogurt, cucumber, mint, dill, black pepper, salt and hot pepper sauce, if desired, in small bowl. Serve burgers on rolls with sauce.

PER SERVING
calories 124
total fat 2g
saturated fat 1g
cholesterol 54mg
sodium 166mg
carbohydrates 21g
dietary fiber 1g
protein 9g

DIETARY EXCHANGES
½ bread/starch,
½ meat, 2½ vegetable

Roasted Chicken Salad

Makes 2 servings

4 cups spring salad greens or mesclun

1 boneless skinless chicken breast (4 ounces), cooked and cut into 1-inch pieces

10 cherry or grape tomatoes, quartered

1 cucumber, sliced

1 red or yellow bell pepper, cut into strips

½ cup sliced red onion

¼ cup reduced-fat, reduced-sodium Italian salad dressing

Black pepper (optional)

1. Combine greens, chicken, tomatoes, cucumber, bell pepper, onion and dressing in large bowl; toss well.

2. Transfer mixture to plate. Season with black pepper, if desired.

PER SERVING
calories 150
total fat 2g
saturated fat 0g
cholesterol 40mg
sodium 450mg
carbohydrates 16g
dietary fiber 4g
protein 16g

DIETARY EXCHANGES
2 meat, 3 vegetable

Sprouts and Bulgur Sandwiches

Makes 4 servings

½ cup bulgur wheat

1 cup water

1 container (8 ounces) plain
low-fat yogurt

¼ cup fat-free salad dressing or
mayonnaise

1½ teaspoons curry powder

1 cup shredded carrots

½ cup chopped apple

⅓ cup coarsely chopped peanuts

2 cups fresh alfalfa sprouts

8 very thin slices wheat bread,
toasted

1. Rinse bulgur under cold running water; drain. Bring 1 cup water to a boil in small saucepan over high heat. Stir in bulgur. Remove from heat. Let stand, uncovered, 20 minutes. Drain well; squeeze out excess liquid.

2. Combine yogurt, salad dressing and curry powder in medium bowl. Stir in bulgur, carrots, apple and peanuts. Cover and refrigerate.

3. Arrange sprouts on 4 slices bread. Spread with bulgur mixture. Top with remaining bread slices.

PER SERVING
calories 274
total fat 9g
saturated fat 2g
cholesterol 3mg
sodium 439mg
carbohydrates 43g
dietary fiber 10g
protein 12g

DIETARY EXCHANGES
2 bread/starch,
½ milk, 1 vegetable,
1½ fat

Chicken Caesar Salad
with Homemade Croutons

Makes 4 servings

- 3 to 4 slices (¾-inch-thick) whole grain artisan bread, cut into ¾-inch cubes (about 2 cups)
- 2 tablespoons olive oil
- 1½ teaspoons salt-free garlic-herb seasoning, divided
- 2 boneless skinless chicken breasts (4 ounces each)
- 8 cups torn romaine lettuce
- ¼ cup fat-free Caesar dressing
- ⅓ cup shredded Parmesan cheese

1. To make croutons, preheat oven to 350°F. Place bread cubes in gallon-size resealable bag. Drizzle with oil and ½ teaspoon seasoning. Seal bag; shake until bread is evenly coated with oil and seasoning. Spread bread cubes in single layer on baking sheet. Bake 12 to 15 minutes, turning 2 or 3 times during baking, until bread is just crisp (bread will continue to crisp as it cools). Remove from oven; set aside.

2. Prepare grill for direct cooking. Season chicken with remaining 1 teaspoon seasoning. Grill chicken over medium heat, covered, about 8 to 10 minutes, turning once, until chicken is no longer pink in center. Remove from grill. Let stand 5 minutes.

3. Meanwhile, in large bowl, toss together lettuce, dressing, cheese and croutons. Divide among four dinner plates. Cut chicken into strips and top each salad with chicken.

Grilled Buffalo Chicken Wraps

Makes 4 servings

- 4 boneless skinless chicken breasts (about 4 ounces each)
- ¼ cup plus 2 tablespoons buffalo wing sauce, divided
- 2 cups broccoli slaw
- 1 tablespoon light blue cheese salad dressing
- 4 (8-inch) whole wheat tortillas, warmed

1. Place chicken in large resealable food storage bag. Add ¼ cup buffalo sauce; seal bag. Marinate in refrigerator 15 minutes.

2. Meanwhile, prepare grill for direct cooking over medium-high heat. Grill chicken 5 to 6 minutes per side or until no longer pink. When cool enough to handle, slice chicken and combine with remaining 2 tablespoons buffalo sauce in medium bowl.

3. Combine broccoli slaw and blue cheese dressing in medium bowl; mix well.

4. Arrange chicken and broccoli slaw evenly down center of each tortilla. Roll up to secure filling. To serve, cut in half diagonally.

Tip: If you don't like the spicy flavor of buffalo wing sauce, substitute your favorite barbecue sauce.

PER SERVING
calories 290
total fat 8g
saturated fat 2g
cholesterol 65mg
sodium 790mg
carbohydrates 25g
dietary fiber 5g
protein 28g

DIETARY EXCHANGES
1 bread/starch,
1 meat, 1 vegetable,
½ fat

Chicken and Ginger Spinach Salad

Makes 4 servings

Dressing

- ⅓ cup fresh orange juice
- 1 tablespoon grated fresh ginger
- 3 tablespoons cider vinegar
- 3 tablespoons pourable sugar substitute*
- 1½ tablespoons canola oil
- ¼ teaspoon red pepper flakes
- ¼ teaspoon salt

Salad

- 2 cups water
- 3 ounces fresh snow peas or sugar snap peas
- 6 ounces baby spinach (about 6 cups)
- 2 ounces sliced red onion (2-inch strips)
- 1 package (8½ ounces) diced cooked chicken breast (about 1¾ cups)
- 2 cups whole strawberries, quartered
- ¼ cup (1 ounce) pistachio nuts or slivered almonds, toasted**

This recipe was tested using sucralose-based sugar substitute.

**To toast pistachios, spread in single layer in heavy skillet. Cook over medium heat 1 to 2 minutes or until nuts are lightly browned, stirring frequently.*

1. Combine dressing ingredients in small jar. Secure with lid; shake until well blended.

2. Bring water to a boil in large saucepan. Add peas; boil 30 seconds. Drain and immediately rinse under cold water to stop the cooking process.

3. To serve, arrange spinach on four plates. Top with onion, chicken, snow peas and strawberries. Sprinkle with nuts. Shake dressing; serve with salad.

Mediterranean Sandwiches

Makes 6 servings

1¼ pounds chicken tenders, cut crosswise in half

1 large tomato, diced

½ small cucumber, halved lengthwise, seeded and sliced

½ cup sweet onion slices (about 1 small)

2 tablespoons cider vinegar

1 tablespoon olive or canola oil

3 teaspoons minced fresh oregano leaves *or* ½ teaspoon dried oregano

2 teaspoons minced fresh mint leaves *or* ¼ teaspoon dried mint

¼ teaspoon salt

12 lettuce leaves (optional)

6 (6-inch) whole wheat pita bread rounds, cut in half crosswise

1. Spray large nonstick skillet with nonstick cooking spray; heat over medium heat. Add chicken; cook and stir 7 to 10 minutes or until browned and cooked through. Let stand 5 to 10 minutes to cool slightly.

2. Combine chicken, tomato, cucumber and onion in medium bowl. Add vinegar, oil, oregano, mint and salt; toss to coat.

3. Place 1 lettuce leaf in each pita bread half, if desired. Divide chicken mixture evenly among pita bread halves.

PER SERVING
calories 242
total fat 6g
saturated fat 1g
cholesterol 50mg
sodium 353mg
carbohydrates 24g
dietary fiber 2g
protein 23g

DIETARY EXCHANGES
1½ bread/starch,
2½ meat

scrumptious soups

Sweet Potato Bisque

Makes 4 servings

1 **pound sweet potatoes, peeled and cut into 2-inch chunks**
2 **teaspoons butter**
½ **cup finely chopped onion**
1 **teaspoon curry powder**
½ **teaspoon ground coriander**
¼ **teaspoon salt**
⅔ **cup unsweetened apple juice**
1 **cup buttermilk**
¼ **cup water (optional)**
    Snipped fresh chives (optional)
    Plain nonfat yogurt (optional)

1. Place sweet potatoes in large saucepan; cover with water. Bring to a boil over high heat. Cook 15 minutes or until potatoes are fork-tender. Drain; cool under cold running water.

2. Meanwhile, melt butter in small saucepan over medium heat. Add onion; cook and stir 2 minutes. Stir in curry powder, coriander and salt; cook and stir 1 minute or until onion is tender. Remove from heat; stir in apple juice.

3. Combine sweet potatoes, buttermilk and onion mixture in food processor or blender; cover and process until smooth. Return to saucepan; stir in ¼ cup water, if necessary, to thin to desired consistency. Cook and stir over medium heat until heated through. ***Do not boil.*** Garnish with chives or dollop of yogurt.

Sausage Vegetable Rotini Soup

Makes 4 servings

1 tablespoon olive oil

6 ounces bulk pork sausage

1 cup chopped onion

1 cup chopped green bell pepper

3 cups water

1 can (about 14 ounces) reduced-sodium diced tomatoes

¼ cup ketchup

2 teaspoons reduced-sodium beef bouillon granules

2 teaspoons chili powder

4 ounces uncooked tri-colored rotini pasta

1 cup frozen corn, thawed and drained

1. Heat oil in large saucepan over medium-high heat. Add sausage; cook 3 minutes or until no longer pink, stirring to break up sausage. Drain fat. Add onion and bell pepper; cook and stir 3 to 4 minutes or until onion is translucent.

2. Add water, tomatoes, ketchup, bouillon and chili powder; bring to a boil over high heat. Stir in pasta; return to a boil. Reduce heat to medium-low; simmer, uncovered, 12 minutes. Stir in corn; cook 2 minutes or until pasta is tender and corn is heated through.

PER SERVING
calories 311
total fat 9g
saturated fat 2g
cholesterol 31mg
sodium 272mg
carbohydrates 45g
dietary fiber 4g
protein 14g

DIETARY EXCHANGES
2½ bread/starch,
1 meat, ½ vegetable,
1 fat

Chickpea-Vegetable Soup

Makes 4 servings

- 1 teaspoon olive oil
- 1 cup chopped onion
- ½ cup chopped green bell pepper
- 2 cloves garlic, minced
- 2 cans (about 14 ounces each) no-salt-added chopped tomatoes
- 3 cups water
- 2 cups broccoli florets
- 1 can (about 15 ounces) chickpeas, rinsed, drained and slightly mashed
- ½ cup (3 ounces) uncooked orzo or rosamarina pasta
- 1 whole bay leaf
- 1 tablespoon chopped fresh thyme *or* 1 teaspoon dried thyme
- 1 tablespoon chopped fresh rosemary leaves *or* 1 teaspoon dried rosemary
- 1 tablespoon lime or lemon juice
- ½ teaspoon ground turmeric
- ¼ teaspoon salt
- ¼ teaspoon ground red pepper
- ¼ cup pumpkin seeds or sunflower kernels

1. Heat oil in large saucepan over medium heat. Add onion, bell pepper and garlic; cook and stir 5 minutes or until vegetables are tender.

2. Add tomatoes, water, broccoli, chickpeas, orzo, bay leaf, thyme, rosemary, lime juice, turmeric, salt and ground red pepper. Bring to a boil over high heat. Reduce heat to medium-low; cover and simmer 10 to 12 minutes or until orzo is tender.

3. Remove and discard bay leaf. Ladle soup into four serving bowls; sprinkle with pumpkin seeds.

Middle Eastern Lentil Soup

Makes 4 servings

1 cup dried lentils

2 tablespoons olive oil

1 small onion, chopped

1 medium red bell pepper, chopped

1 teaspoon whole fennel seeds

½ teaspoon ground cumin

¼ teaspoon ground red pepper

4 cups water

½ teaspoon salt

1 tablespoon lemon juice

½ cup plain low-fat yogurt

2 tablespoons chopped fresh parsley

1. Rinse lentils, discarding any debris or blemished lentils; drain.

2. Heat oil in large saucepan over medium-high heat until hot. Add onion and bell pepper; cook and stir 5 minutes or until tender. Add fennel seeds, cumin and ground red pepper; cook and stir 1 minute.

3. Add water, lentils and salt. Bring to a boil. Reduce heat to low. Cover and simmer 25 to 30 minutes or until lentils are tender. Stir in lemon juice.

4. To serve, ladle soup into four individual bowls and top with yogurt; sprinkle with parsley.

PER SERVING
calories 266
total fat 8g
saturated fat 1g
cholesterol 2mg
sodium 320mg
carbohydrates 35g
dietary fiber 16g
protein 16g

DIETARY EXCHANGES
2 bread/starch,
1 meat, 1 vegetable,
1 fat

Vegetable-Chicken Noodle Soup

Makes 6 servings

1 cup chopped celery

½ cup thinly sliced leek (white part only)

½ cup chopped carrot

½ cup chopped turnip

6 cups fat-free reduced-sodium chicken broth, divided

1 tablespoon minced fresh parsley

1½ teaspoons fresh thyme *or* ½ teaspoon dried thyme

1 teaspoon minced fresh rosemary leaves *or* ¼ teaspoon dried rosemary

1 teaspoon balsamic vinegar

¼ teaspoon black pepper

2 ounces uncooked yolk-free wide noodles

1 cup boneless skinless chicken breast, cooked and diced

1. Combine celery, leek, carrot, turnip and ⅓ cup broth in large saucepan; cover and cook over medium heat 12 to 15 minutes or until vegetables are tender, stirring occasionally.

2. Stir in remaining 5⅔ cups broth, parsley, thyme, rosemary, vinegar and pepper; bring to a boil over medium-high heat. Stir in noodles; cook until noodles are tender.

3. Stir in chicken. Reduce heat to medium; cook until heated through.

PER SERVING
calories 98
total fat 2g
saturated fat 1g
cholesterol 18mg
sodium 73mg
carbohydrates 12g
dietary fiber 1g
protein 10g

DIETARY EXCHANGES
½ bread/starch,
1 meat, ½ vegetable

Ground Beef, Spinach and Barley Soup

Makes 4 servings

12 ounces 95% lean ground beef

4 cups water

1 can (about 14 ounces) stewed tomatoes

1½ cups thinly sliced carrots

1 cup chopped onion

½ cup uncooked quick-cooking barley

1½ teaspoons beef bouillon granules

1½ teaspoons dried thyme

1 teaspoon dried oregano

½ teaspoon garlic powder

¼ teaspoon black pepper

⅛ teaspoon salt

3 cups fresh spinach leaves

1. Brown beef in large saucepan over medium-high heat 6 to 8 minutes, stirring to break up meat. Rinse beef under warm water; drain.

2. Return beef to saucepan; stir in 4 cups water, tomatoes, carrots, onion, barley, bouillon, thyme, oregano, garlic powder, pepper and salt; bring to a boil over high heat.

3. Reduce heat to medium-low. Cover; simmer 12 to 15 minutes or until barley and vegetables are tender, stirring occasionally. Stir in spinach; cook until spinach starts to wilt.

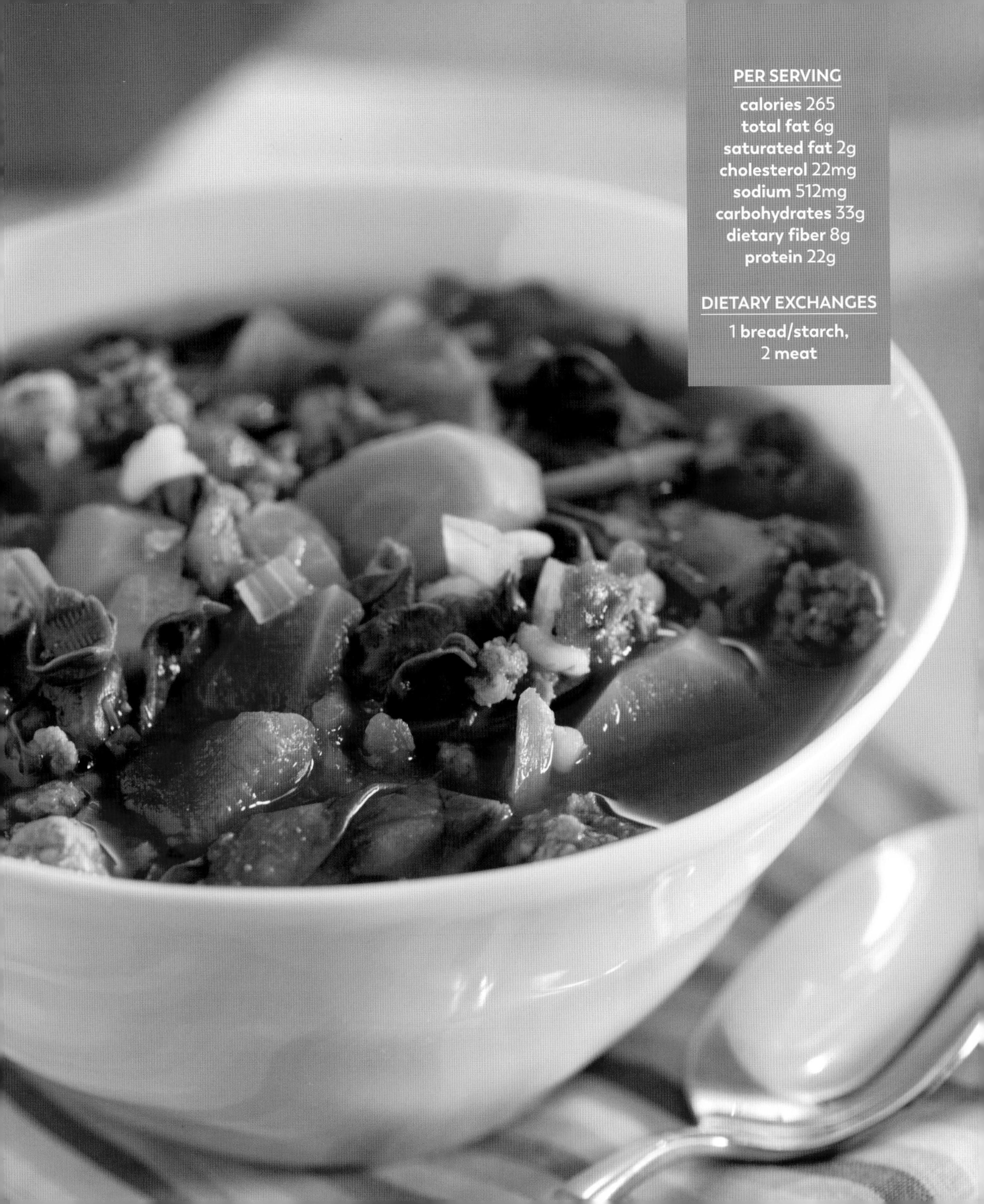

PER SERVING

calories 265
total fat 6g
saturated fat 2g
cholesterol 22mg
sodium 512mg
carbohydrates 33g
dietary fiber 8g
protein 22g

DIETARY EXCHANGES

1 **bread/starch,**
2 **meat**

Black and White Chili

Makes 6 servings

- 1 pound chicken tenders, cut into ¾-inch pieces
- 1 cup coarsely chopped onion
- 1 can (about 15 ounces) Great Northern beans, drained
- 1 can (about 15 ounces) black beans, drained
- 1 can (about 14 ounces) Mexican-style stewed tomatoes, undrained
- 2 tablespoons Texas-style chili powder seasoning mix

Slow Cooker Directions

1. Spray large skillet with nonstick cooking spray; heat over medium heat until hot. Add chicken and onion; cook and stir 5 minutes or until chicken is browned.

2. Combine chicken mixture, beans, tomatoes with juice and chili seasoning in slow cooker. Cover; cook on LOW 4 to 4½ hours.

Serving Suggestion: For a change of pace, this delicious chili is excellent served over cooked rice or pasta.

PER SERVING
calories 260
total fat 2g
saturated fat 1g
cholesterol 44mg
sodium 403mg
carbohydrates 34g
dietary fiber 8g
protein 27g

DIETARY EXCHANGES
2 bread/starch,
2 meat

Slow Cooker Veggie Stew

Makes 4 to 6 servings

- **1** tablespoon vegetable oil
- **⅔** cup carrot slices
- **½** cup diced onion
- **2** cloves garlic, chopped
- **2** cans (about 14 ounces each) vegetable broth
- **1½** cups chopped green cabbage
- **½** cup cut green beans
- **½** cup diced zucchini
- **1** tablespoon tomato paste
- **½** teaspoon dried basil
- **½** teaspoon dried oregano
- **¼** teaspoon salt

Slow Cooker Directions

1. Heat oil in medium skillet over medium-high heat. Add carrot, onion and garlic; cook and stir until tender. Transfer to slow cooker.

2. Stir in remaining ingredients. Cover; cook on LOW 8 to 10 hours or on HIGH 4 to 5 hours.

PER SERVING
calories 83
total fat 4g
saturated fat 1g
cholesterol 0mg
sodium 654mg
carbohydrates 10g
dietary fiber 2g
protein 3g

DIETARY EXCHANGES
2 vegetable,
1 fat

Tuscan Chicken with White Beans

Makes 4 servings

1 large bulb fennel (about ¾ pound)

1 teaspoon olive oil

1 teaspoon dried rosemary

½ teaspoon black pepper

½ pound boneless skinless chicken thighs, cut into ¾-inch pieces

1 can (about 14 ounces) no-salt-added stewed tomatoes, undrained

1 can (about 14 ounces) fat-free reduced-sodium chicken broth

1 can (about 15 ounces) cannellini beans, rinsed and drained

Hot pepper sauce (optional)

1. Cut off and reserve ¼ cup chopped feathery fennel tops. Chop bulb into ½-inch pieces. Heat oil in large saucepan over medium heat. Add chopped fennel bulb; cook 5 minutes, stirring occasionally.

2. Sprinkle rosemary and pepper over chicken; add to saucepan. Cook and stir 2 minutes. Add tomatoes with juice and broth; bring to a boil. Reduce heat; simmer, covered, 10 minutes. Stir in beans; simmer, uncovered, 15 minutes or until chicken is cooked through and sauce thickens. Season to taste with hot pepper sauce. Ladle into four shallow bowls; top with reserved fennel tops.

PER SERVING
calories 215
total fat 6g
saturated fat 2g
cholesterol 34mg
sodium 321mg
carbohydrates 24g
dietary fiber 7g
protein 17g

DIETARY EXCHANGES
1 bread/starch,
2 meat, 1½ vegetable

Caribbean Callaloo Soup

Makes 6 servings

1 teaspoon olive oil

1 large onion, chopped

4 cloves garlic, minced

¾ pound boneless skinless chicken breasts, thinly sliced crosswise

1½ pounds butternut squash, cut into ½-inch cubes

3 cans (about 14 ounces each) fat-free reduced-sodium chicken broth

2 jalapeño peppers,* seeded and minced

2 teaspoons dried thyme

½ (10-ounce) package fresh spinach, stemmed and torn

¼ cup plus 2 tablespoons shredded sweetened coconut, toasted**

Jalapeño peppers can sting and irritate the skin, so wear rubber gloves when handling peppers and do not touch your eyes.

**To toast coconut, spread in a single layer in heavy-bottomed skillet. Cook and stir 1 to 2 minutes or until lightly browned. Remove from skillet immediately.*

1. Heat oil in large nonstick skillet over medium-low heat. Add onion and garlic; cook and stir 5 minutes or until onion is tender. Add chicken; cover and cook 5 to 7 minutes or until chicken is no longer pink in center.

2. Add squash, broth, jalapeño peppers and thyme; bring to a boil over medium-high heat. Reduce heat to low. Simmer, covered, 15 to 20 minutes or until squash is very tender.

3. Remove skillet from heat; stir in spinach until wilted. Ladle into bowls and sprinkle with toasted coconut.

PER SERVING
calories 255
total fat 5g
saturated fat 2g
cholesterol 24mg
sodium 580mg
carbohydrates 36g
dietary fiber 4g
protein 15g

DIETARY EXCHANGES
2 bread/starch,
1 meat, 1 vegetable,
½ fat

effortless entrées

Turkey Sausage & Spinach Stuffed Shells

Makes 6 servings (3 filled shells per serving)

18 uncooked jumbo shell pasta

1 teaspoon olive oil

8 ounces spicy Italian turkey sausage, casings removed

½ cup chopped onion

2 cloves garlic, minced

1 package (6 ounces) baby spinach

1 cup fat-free ricotta cheese

1½ cups tomato-basil pasta sauce, divided

½ cup shredded Parmesan cheese, divided

¼ cup chopped fresh basil

1. Preheat oven to 375°F. Cook pasta according to package directions; drain.

2. Meanwhile, heat oil in large nonstick skillet over medium heat. Add sausage, onion and garlic; cook 5 minutes or until sausage begins to brown, stirring to break up meat. Add spinach in batches; cook and stir until wilted. Remove from heat; stir in ricotta cheese, ½ cup pasta sauce and ¼ cup Parmesan cheese.

3. Arrange shells in 2-quart casserole. Fill shells evenly with turkey mixture. Spoon remaining 1 cup pasta sauce evenly over shells. Cover with foil.

4. Bake 30 to 35 minutes or until heated through. Top with remaining ¼ cup Parmesan cheese and basil.

Chicken Mirabella

Makes 4 servings

4 boneless skinless chicken breasts (about 4 ounces each)

½ cup pitted prunes

½ cup assorted pitted olives (black, green and/or a combination)

¼ cup light white grape juice or dry white wine

2 tablespoons olive oil

1 tablespoon capers

1 tablespoon red wine vinegar

1 teaspoon dried oregano

1 clove garlic, minced

½ teaspoon chopped fresh parsley, plus additional for garnish

2 teaspoons packed brown sugar

1. Preheat oven to 350°F.

2. Place chicken in 8-inch baking dish. Combine prunes, olives, grape juice, oil, capers, vinegar, oregano, garlic and ½ teaspoon parsley in medium bowl. Pour evenly over chicken. Sprinkle with brown sugar.

3. Bake 25 to 30 minutes or until chicken is no longer pink in center, basting with sauce halfway through cooking. Garnish with additional parsley.

Tip: For more intense flavor, marinate chicken at least 8 hours or overnight and sprinkle with brown sugar just before baking.

Serving Suggestion: Serve with long grain and wild rice.

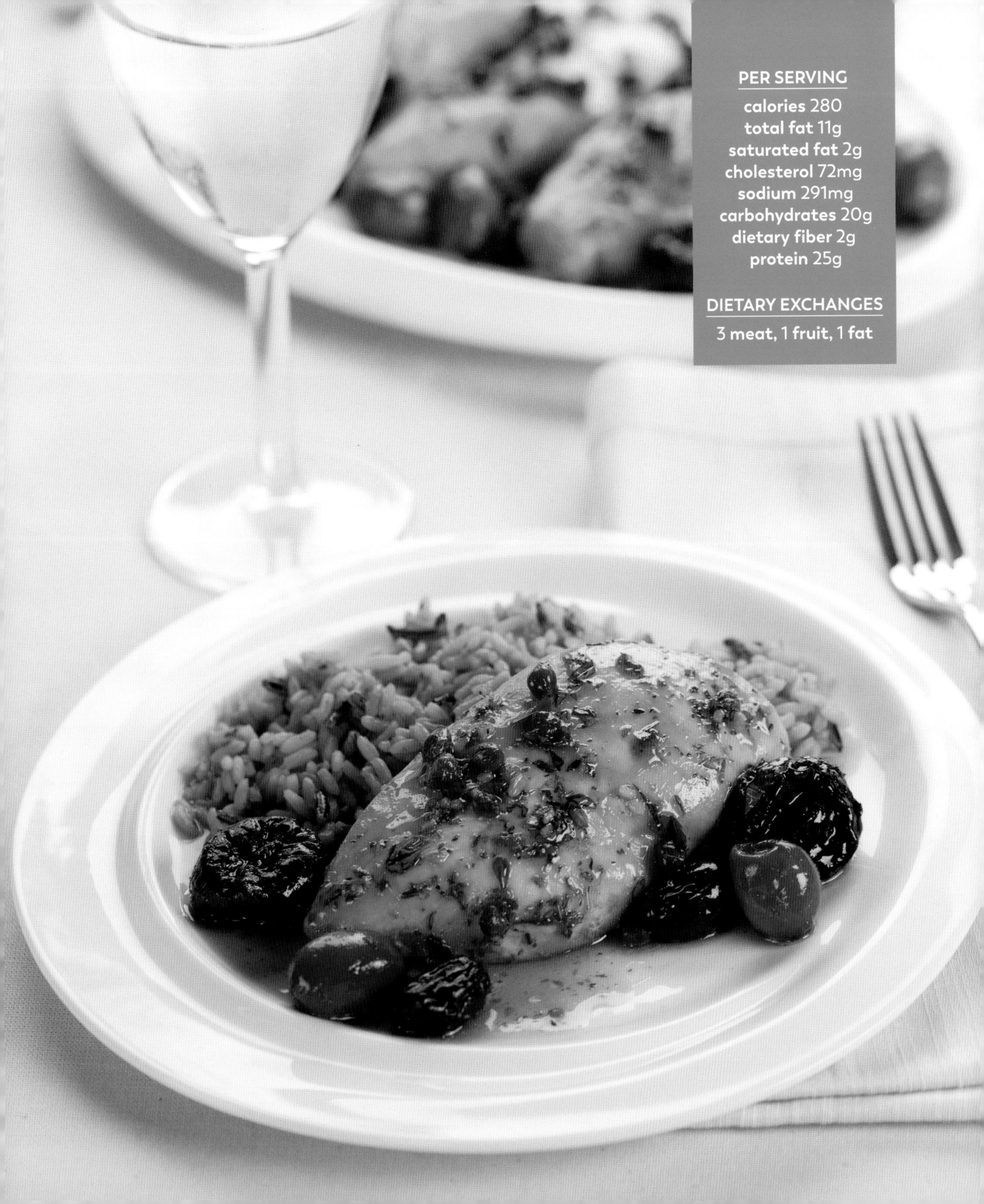

PER SERVING

calories 280
total fat 11g
saturated fat 2g
cholesterol 72mg
sodium 291mg
carbohydrates 20g
dietary fiber 2g
protein 25g

DIETARY EXCHANGES

3 meat, 1 fruit, 1 fat

Stir-Fried Beef & Spinach

Makes 2 servings

1 package (6 ounces) fresh
   spinach, stemmed and torn

⅛ teaspoon salt

8 ounces boneless beef top
   sirloin steak, thinly sliced

¼ cup stir-fry sauce

1 teaspoon sugar

½ teaspoon curry powder

¼ teaspoon ground ginger

1. Spray large skillet or wok with nonstick cooking spray; heat over high heat. Add spinach; stir-fry 1 minute or until wilted. Transfer spinach to serving platter. Sprinkle with salt; keep warm.

2. Spray same skillet with cooking spray; heat over high heat. Add beef; stir-fry 2 minutes or until barely pink. Add stir-fry sauce, sugar, curry powder and ginger; cook and stir 1½ minutes or until sauce thickens. Serve with spinach.

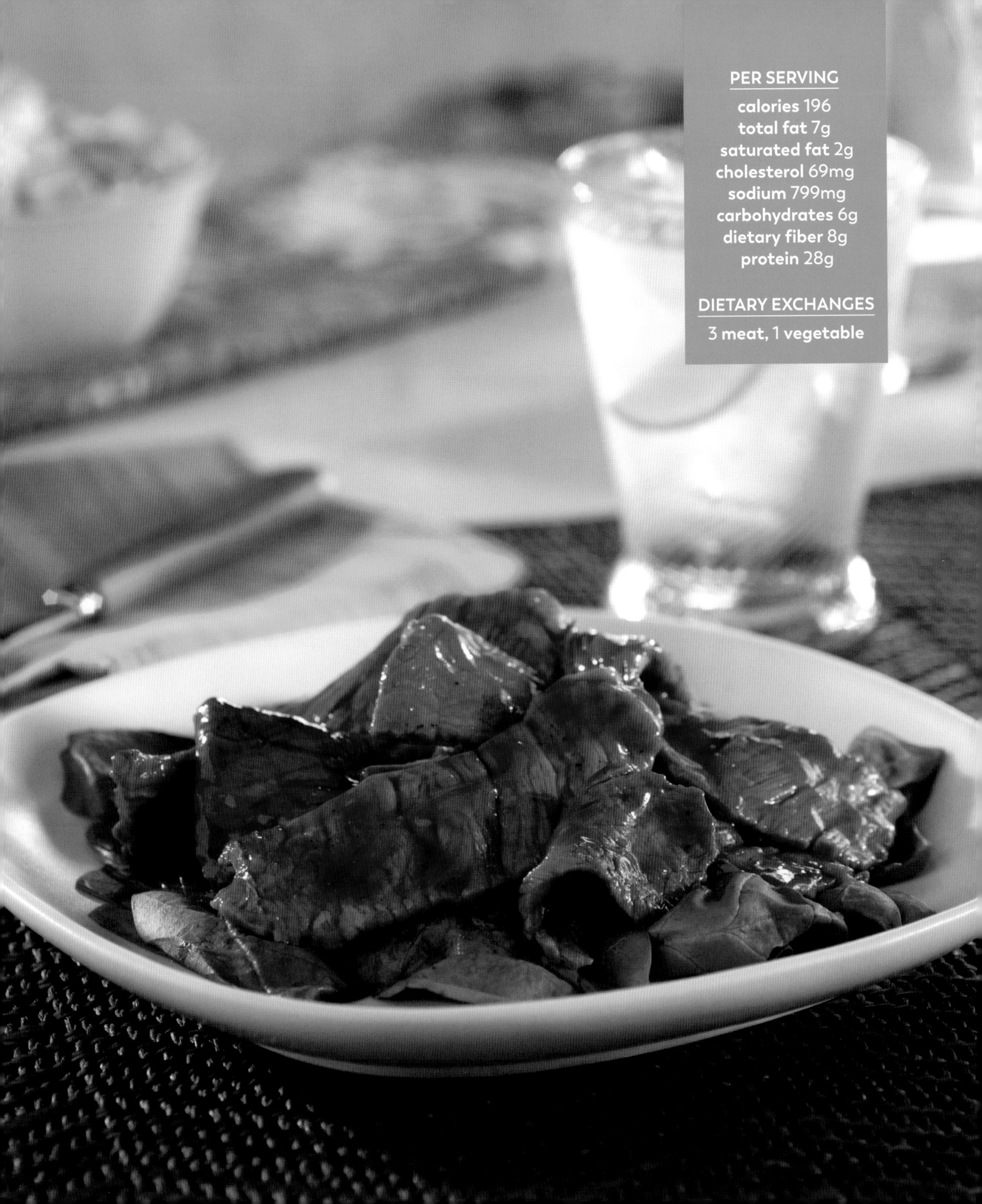

PER SERVING

calories 196
total fat 7g
saturated fat 2g
cholesterol 69mg
sodium 799mg
carbohydrates 6g
dietary fiber 8g
protein 28g

DIETARY EXCHANGES

3 meat, 1 vegetable

Lemon-Garlic Salmon with Tzatziki Sauce

Makes 4 servings

½ cup diced cucumber

¾ teaspoon salt, divided

1 cup plain nonfat Greek yogurt

2 tablespoons fresh lemon juice, divided

1 teaspoon grated lemon peel, divided

1 teaspoon minced garlic, divided

¼ teaspoon black pepper

4 (4-ounce) skinless salmon fillets

1. Place cucumber in small colander set over small bowl; sprinkle with ¼ teaspoon salt. Drain 1 hour.

2. For tzatziki sauce, stir yogurt, cucumber, 1 tablespoon lemon juice, ½ teaspoon lemon peel, ½ teaspoon garlic and ¼ teaspoon salt in small bowl until combined. Cover and refrigerate until ready to use.

3. Combine remaining 1 tablespoon lemon juice, ½ teaspoon lemon peel, ½ teaspoon garlic, ¼ teaspoon salt and pepper in small bowl; mix well. Rub evenly onto salmon.

4. Heat nonstick grill pan over medium-high heat. Cook salmon 5 minutes per side or until fish begins to flake when tested with fork. Serve with tzatziki sauce.

Serving Suggestion: Serve this Mediterranean-inspired dish with fresh vegetables or a savory salad, if desired.

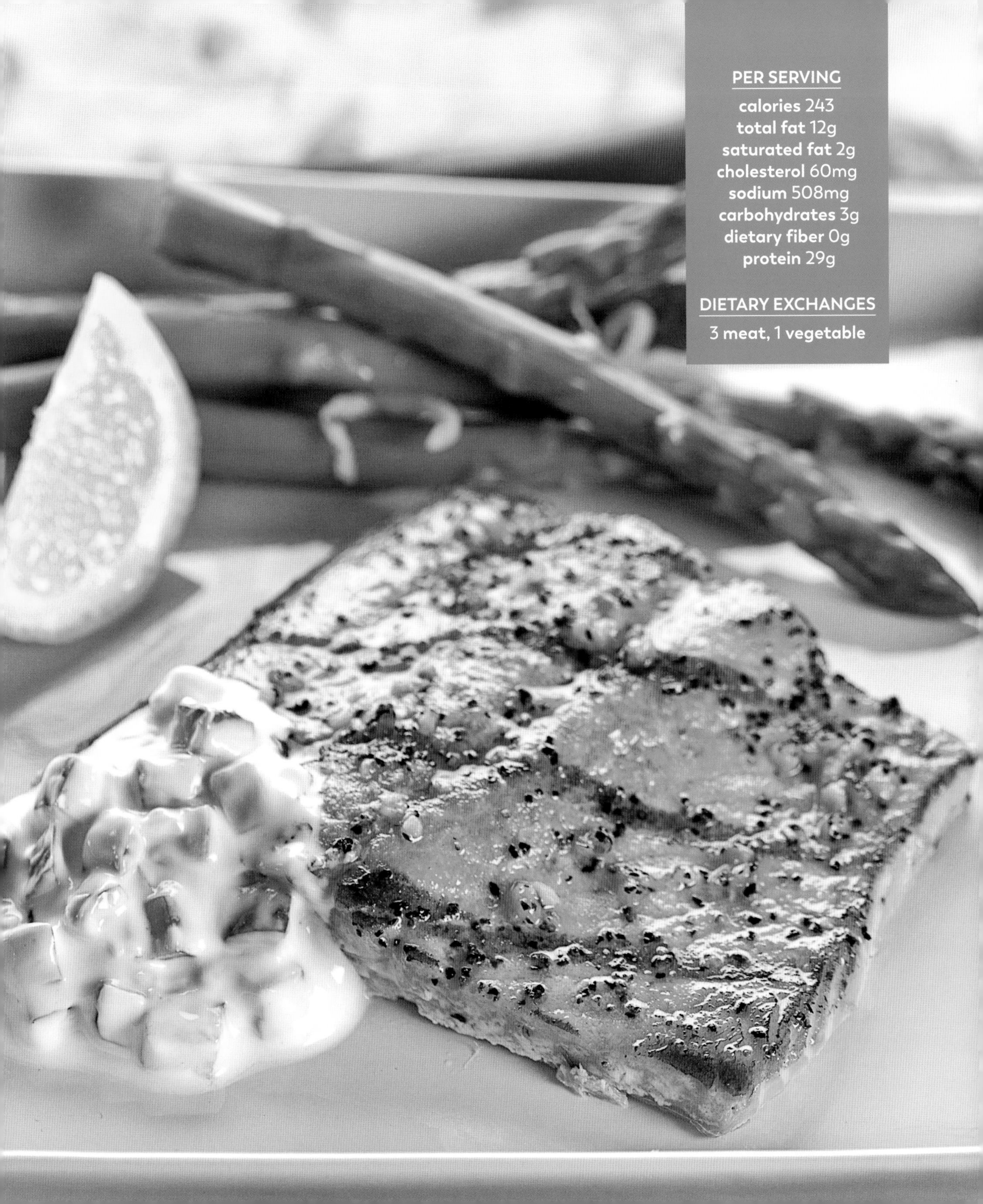

PER SERVING

calories 243
total fat 12g
saturated fat 2g
cholesterol 60mg
sodium 508mg
carbohydrates 3g
dietary fiber 0g
protein 29g

DIETARY EXCHANGES

3 meat, 1 vegetable

Sweet and Sour Chicken

Makes 4 servings

- 2 tablespoons unseasoned rice vinegar
- 2 tablespoons reduced-sodium soy sauce
- 3 cloves garlic, minced
- ½ teaspoon minced fresh ginger
- ¼ teaspoon red pepper flakes (optional)
- 6 ounces boneless skinless chicken breasts, cut into ½-inch strips
- 1 teaspoon vegetable oil
- 3 green onions, cut into 1-inch pieces
- 1 large green bell pepper, cut into 1-inch pieces
- 1 tablespoon cornstarch
- ½ cup fat-free reduced-sodium chicken broth
- 2 tablespoons apricot fruit spread
- 1 can (11 ounces) mandarin orange segments, drained
- 2 cups hot cooked white rice

1. Whisk vinegar, soy sauce, garlic, ginger and red pepper flakes, if desired, in medium bowl until smooth and well blended. Add chicken; toss to coat. Marinate 20 minutes at room temperature.

2. Heat oil in wok or large nonstick skillet over medium heat. Drain chicken; reserve marinade. Add chicken to wok; stir-fry 3 minutes. Stir in green onions and bell pepper.

3. Stir cornstarch into reserved marinade until well blended. Stir broth, fruit spread and marinade mixture into wok. Bring to a boil; cook and stir 2 minutes or until chicken is cooked through and sauce is thickened. Add oranges; cook until heated through. Serve over rice.

PER SERVING
calories 256
total fat 2g
saturated fat 1g
cholesterol 17mg
sodium 320mg
carbohydrates 37g
dietary fiber 1g
protein 14g

DIETARY EXCHANGES
2 bread/starch,
1 meat, 1 vegetable,
½ fruit

Skillet Fish with Lemon Tarragon "Butter"

Makes 2 servings

2 teaspoons margarine

4 teaspoons lemon juice, divided

½ teaspoon grated lemon peel

¼ teaspoon prepared mustard

¼ teaspoon dried tarragon

⅛ teaspoon salt

2 lean white fish fillets (4 ounces each),* rinsed and patted dry

¼ teaspoon paprika

Cod, orange roughy, flounder, haddock, halibut and sole can be used.

1. Combine margarine, 2 teaspoons lemon juice, lemon peel, mustard, tarragon and salt in small bowl; mix well with fork.

2. Spray 12-inch nonstick skillet with nonstick cooking spray; heat over medium heat. Drizzle fish with remaining 2 teaspoons lemon juice; sprinkle one side of each fillet with paprika.

3. Place fish in skillet, paprika side down; cook 3 minutes. Gently turn and cook 3 minutes longer or until fish is opaque in center and begins to flake when tested with fork. Top with margarine mixture.

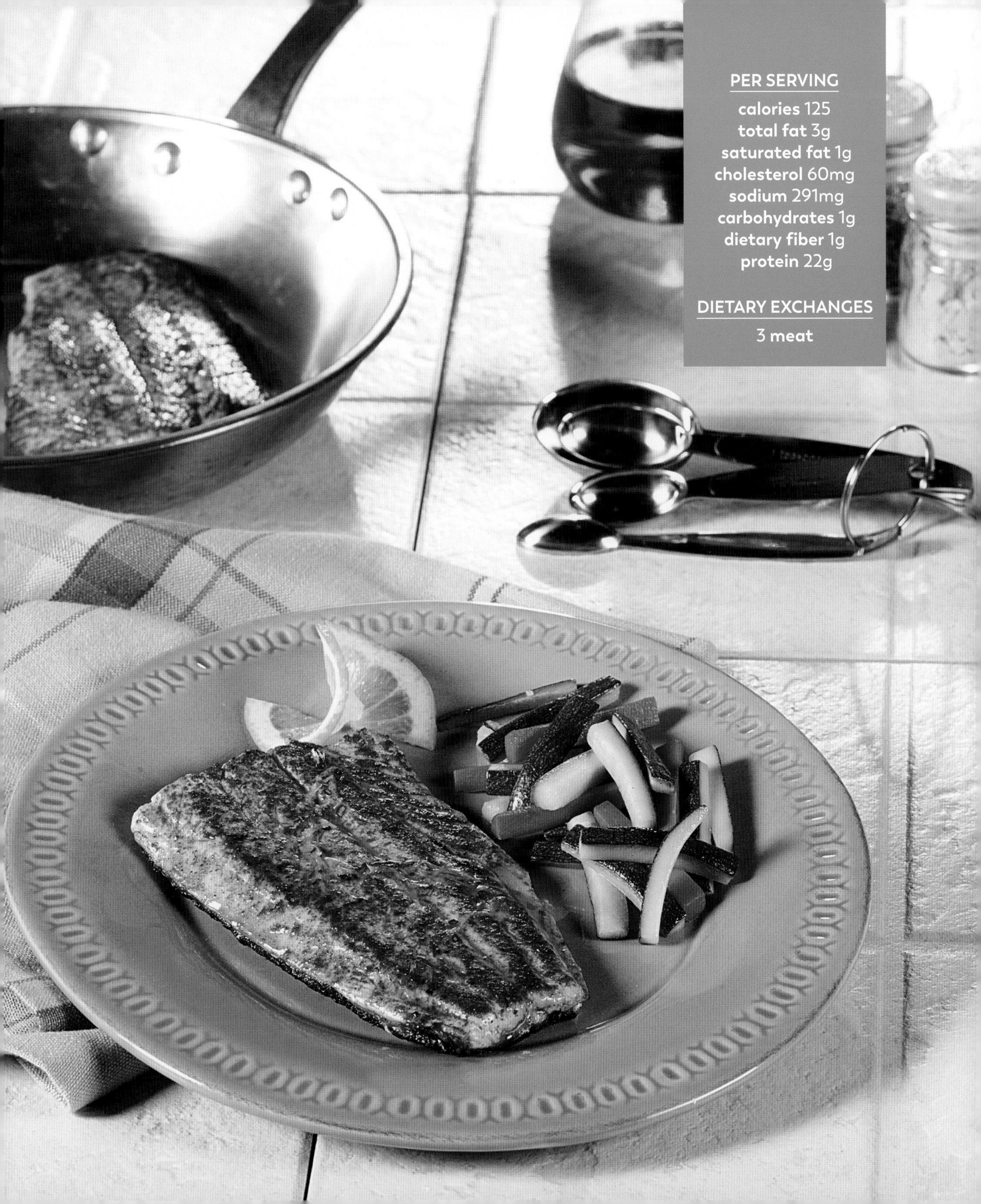

Apple-Cherry Glazed Pork Chops

Makes 4 servings

½ to 1 teaspoon dried thyme

¼ teaspoon salt

¼ teaspoon black pepper

4 boneless pork loin chops
   (3 ounces each), trimmed
   of fat

1⅓ cups unsweetened apple juice

1 small apple, sliced

4 tablespoons sliced green
   onions

4 tablespoons dried tart cherries

2 tablespoons water

2 teaspoons cornstarch

Slow Cooker Directions

1. Combine thyme, salt and pepper in small bowl. Rub onto both sides of pork chops. Spray large nonstick skillet with nonstick olive oil cooking spray and brown both sides of pork on medium-high heat, cooking in batches, if necessary. Transfer to slow cooker.

2. Add apple juice, apple slices, green onions and cherries to same skillet. Simmer, uncovered, 2 to 3 minutes or until apple and green onions are tender. Blend water and cornstarch in small bowl until smooth; stir into skillet. Bring to a boil; cook and stir until thickened. Spoon over pork chops.

3. Cover; cook on LOW 3½ to 4 hours or until pork chops are tender. To serve, spoon fruit and cooking liquid over pork chops.

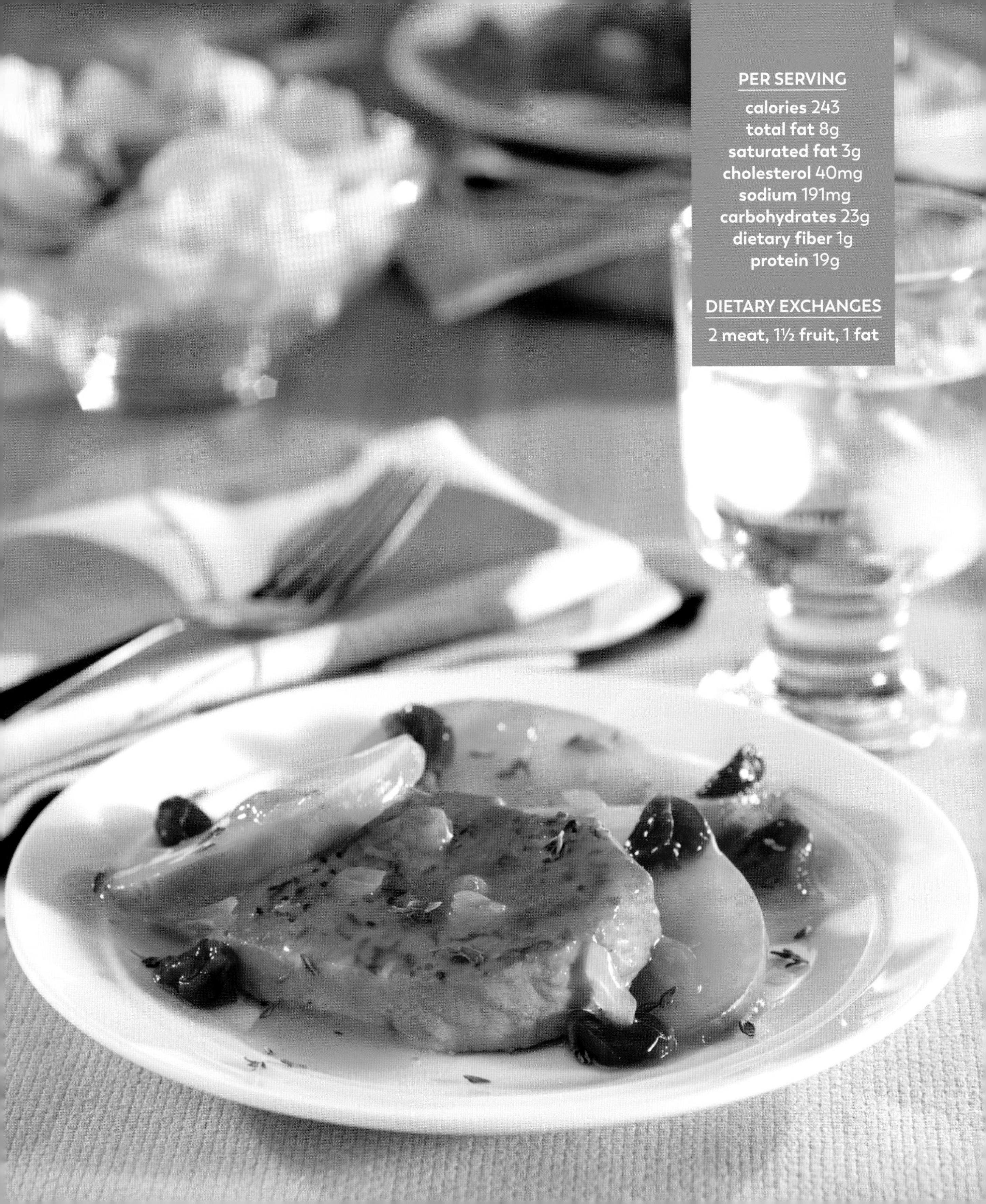

PER SERVING

calories 243
total fat 8g
saturated fat 3g
cholesterol 40mg
sodium 191mg
carbohydrates 23g
dietary fiber 1g
protein 19g

DIETARY EXCHANGES

2 meat, 1½ fruit, 1 fat

Kale & Mushroom Stuffed Chicken Breasts

Makes 4 servings

3 teaspoons olive oil, divided

1 cup coarsely chopped mushrooms

2 cups thinly sliced kale

1 tablespoon fresh lemon juice

½ teaspoon salt, divided

4 boneless skinless chicken breasts (about 4 ounces each)

¼ cup crumbled fat-free feta cheese

¼ teaspoon black pepper

1. Heat 1 teaspoon oil in large skillet over medium-high heat. Add mushrooms; cook and stir 5 minutes or until mushrooms begin to brown. Add kale; cook and stir 8 minutes or until wilted. Sprinkle with lemon juice and ¼ teaspoon salt. Remove to small bowl. Let stand 5 to 10 minutes to cool slightly.

2. Meanwhile, place each chicken breast between sheets of plastic wrap. Pound with meat mallet or rolling pin to about ½-inch thickness.

3. Gently stir feta cheese into mushroom and kale mixture. Spoon ¼ cup mixture down center of each chicken breast. Roll up to enclose filling; secure with toothpicks. Sprinkle with remaining ¼ teaspoon salt and pepper.

4. Wipe out same skillet with paper towels. Add remaining 2 teaspoons oil to skillet; heat over medium heat. Add chicken; brown on all sides. Cover and cook 5 minutes per side or until no longer pink. Remove toothpicks before serving.

Serving Suggestion: Serve this flavorful entrée with a fresh salad or summer vegetables.

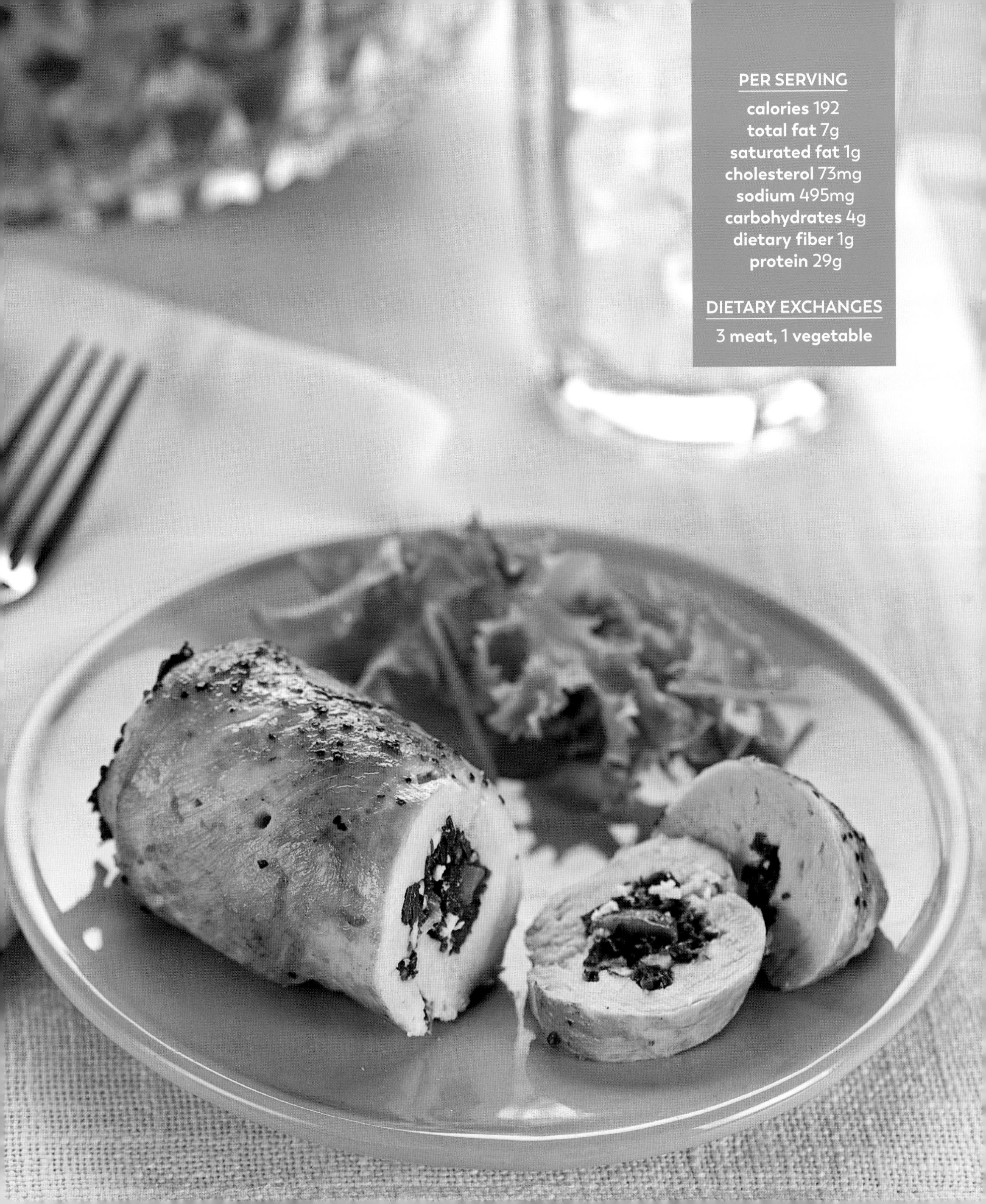

PER SERVING

calories 192
total fat 7g
saturated fat 1g
cholesterol 73mg
sodium 495mg
carbohydrates 4g
dietary fiber 1g
protein 29g

DIETARY EXCHANGES

3 meat, 1 vegetable

Baked Fish with Tomatoes & Herbs

Makes 4 servings

- 4 lean white fish fillets (about 1 pound), such as orange roughy or sole
- 2 tablespoons plus 2 teaspoons lemon juice, divided
- ½ teaspoon paprika
- 1 cup finely chopped seeded tomatoes
- 2 tablespoons capers, rinsed and drained
- 2 tablespoons finely chopped fresh parsley
- 1½ teaspoons dried basil
- 2 teaspoons olive oil
- ¼ teaspoon salt

1. Preheat oven to 350°F. Coat 12×8-inch glass baking pan with nonstick cooking spray.

2. Arrange fish fillets in pan. Drizzle 2 tablespoons lemon juice over fillets; sprinkle with paprika. Cover with foil; bake 18 minutes or until opaque in center and flakes easily when tested with fork.

3. Meanwhile, in medium saucepan, combine tomatoes, capers, parsley, remaining 2 teaspoons lemon juice, basil, oil and salt. Five minutes before fish is done, place saucepan over high heat. Bring to a boil. Reduce heat and simmer 2 minutes or until hot. Remove from heat.

4. Serve fish topped with tomato mixture.

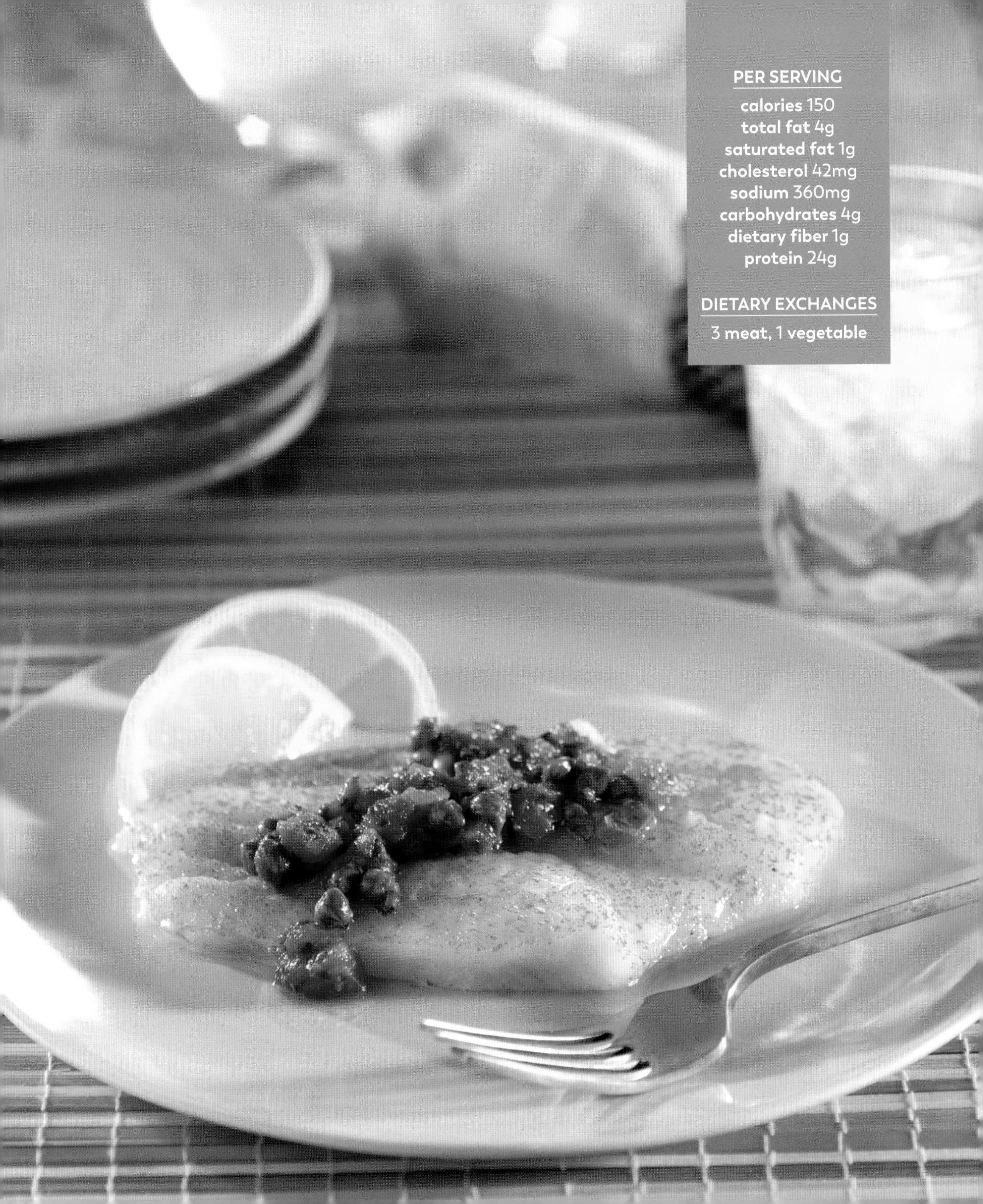

PER SERVING

calories 150
total fat 4g
saturated fat 1g
cholesterol 42mg
sodium 360mg
carbohydrates 4g
dietary fiber 1g
protein 24g

DIETARY EXCHANGES

3 meat, 1 vegetable

Chicken Piccata

Makes 4 servings

3 tablespoons all-purpose flour

½ teaspoon salt

¼ teaspoon black pepper

4 boneless skinless chicken breasts (4 ounces each)

2 teaspoons olive oil

1 teaspoon butter

2 cloves garlic, minced

¾ cup fat-free reduced-sodium chicken broth

1 tablespoon fresh lemon juice

2 tablespoons chopped fresh Italian parsley

1 tablespoon capers, drained

1. Combine flour, salt and pepper in shallow dish. Reserve 1 tablespoon flour mixture for sauce.

2. Pound chicken to ½-inch thickness between sheets of waxed paper with flat side of meat mallet or rolling pin. Coat chicken with remaining flour mixture, shaking off excess.

3. Heat oil and butter in large nonstick skillet over medium heat. Add chicken; cook 4 to 5 minutes per side or until no longer pink in center. Transfer to serving platter; cover loosely with foil.

4. Add garlic to skillet; cook and stir 1 minute. Add reserved flour mixture; cook and stir 1 minute. Add broth and lemon juice; cook 2 minutes or until sauce thickens, stirring frequently. Stir in parsley and capers; spoon sauce over chicken.

PER SERVING
calories 194
total fat 6g
saturated fat 2g
cholesterol 71mg
sodium 473mg
carbohydrates 5g
dietary fiber 1g
protein 27g

DIETARY EXCHANGES
½ bread/starch,
3 meat

Zesty Skillet Pork Chops

Makes 4 servings

- 1 teaspoon chili powder
- ½ teaspoon salt, divided
- 4 lean boneless pork chops (about 1¼ pounds), well trimmed
- 2 cups diced tomatoes
- 1 cup chopped green, red or yellow bell pepper
- ¾ cup thinly sliced celery
- ½ cup chopped onion
- 1 teaspoon dried thyme
- 1 tablespoon hot pepper sauce
- 2 tablespoons finely chopped fresh parsley

1. Rub chili powder and ¼ teaspoon salt evenly over one side of pork chops.

2. Combine tomatoes, bell peppers, celery, onion, thyme and hot pepper sauce in medium bowl; mix well.

3. Lightly spray large nonstick skillet with nonstick cooking spray; heat over medium-high heat. Add pork, seasoned side down; cook 1 minute. Turn pork. Top with tomato mixture; bring to a boil. Reduce heat to low. Cover; cook 25 minutes or until pork is tender and tomato mixture has thickened.

4. Transfer pork to serving plates. Bring tomato mixture to a boil over high heat; cook 2 minutes or until most liquid has evaporated. Remove from heat; stir in parsley and remaining ¼ teaspoon salt. Spoon sauce over pork.

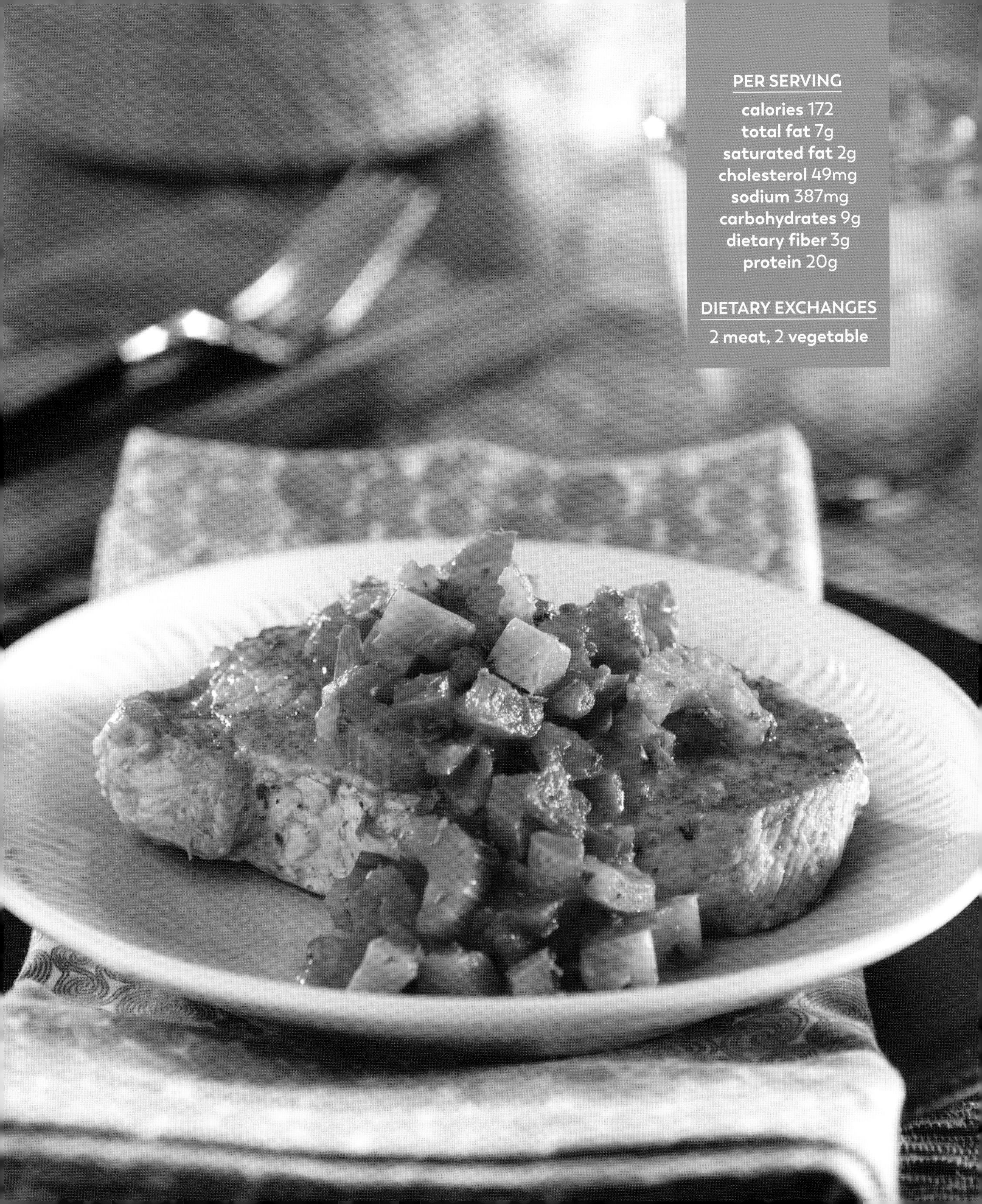

PER SERVING

calories 172
total fat 7g
saturated fat 2g
cholesterol 49mg
sodium 387mg
carbohydrates 9g
dietary fiber 3g
protein 20g

DIETARY EXCHANGES

2 meat, 2 vegetable

Thai Grilled Chicken

Makes 4 servings

- 4 boneless skinless chicken breasts (about 1¼ pounds)
- ¼ cup low-sodium soy sauce
- 2 teaspoons minced garlic
- ½ teaspoon red pepper flakes
- 2 tablespoons honey
- 1 tablespoon fresh lime juice

1. Prepare grill for direct cooking over medium heat. Place chicken in shallow baking dish. Combine soy sauce, garlic and red pepper flakes in small bowl. Pour over chicken, turning to coat. Let stand 10 minutes.

2. Meanwhile, combine honey and lime juice in small bowl; blend well. Set aside.

3. Place chicken on grid; brush with marinade. Discard remaining marinade. Grill, covered, 5 minutes. Brush both sides of chicken with honey mixture. Grill 5 minutes more or until chicken is no longer pink in center.

Serving Suggestion: Serve with steamed white rice, grilled vegetables and/or grilled fruit salad.

PER SERVING
calories 140
total fat 1g
saturated fat 1g
cholesterol 53mg
sodium 349mg
carbohydrates 10g
dietary fiber 1g
protein 22g

DIETARY EXCHANGES
3 meat

Scallop and Artichoke Heart Casserole

Makes 4 servings

1 package (9 ounces) frozen artichoke hearts, cooked and drained

1 pound scallops

1 teaspoon canola or vegetable oil

¼ cup chopped red bell pepper

¼ cup sliced green onions

¼ cup all-purpose flour

2 cups low-fat (1%) milk

1 teaspoon dried tarragon

¼ teaspoon salt

¼ teaspoon white pepper

1 tablespoon chopped fresh parsley

Pinch paprika

1. Preheat oven to 350°F.

2. Cut large artichoke hearts lengthwise into halves; arrange in even layer in 8-inch square baking dish.

3. Rinse scallops; pat dry with paper towel. If scallops are large, cut into halves. Arrange scallops evenly over artichokes.

4. Heat oil in medium saucepan over medium-low heat. Add bell pepper and green onions; cook and stir 5 minutes or until tender. Stir in flour. Gradually stir in milk until smooth. Add tarragon, salt and white pepper; cook and stir over medium heat 10 minutes or until sauce boils and thickens. Pour sauce over scallops.

5. Bake, uncovered, 25 minutes or until casserole is bubbly and scallops are opaque. Sprinkle with parsley and paprika before serving.

Tip: White pepper is a mild version of the common black pepper. They both originate from the same berries, which are called peppercorns. White pepper helps to maintain consistent color in light foods.

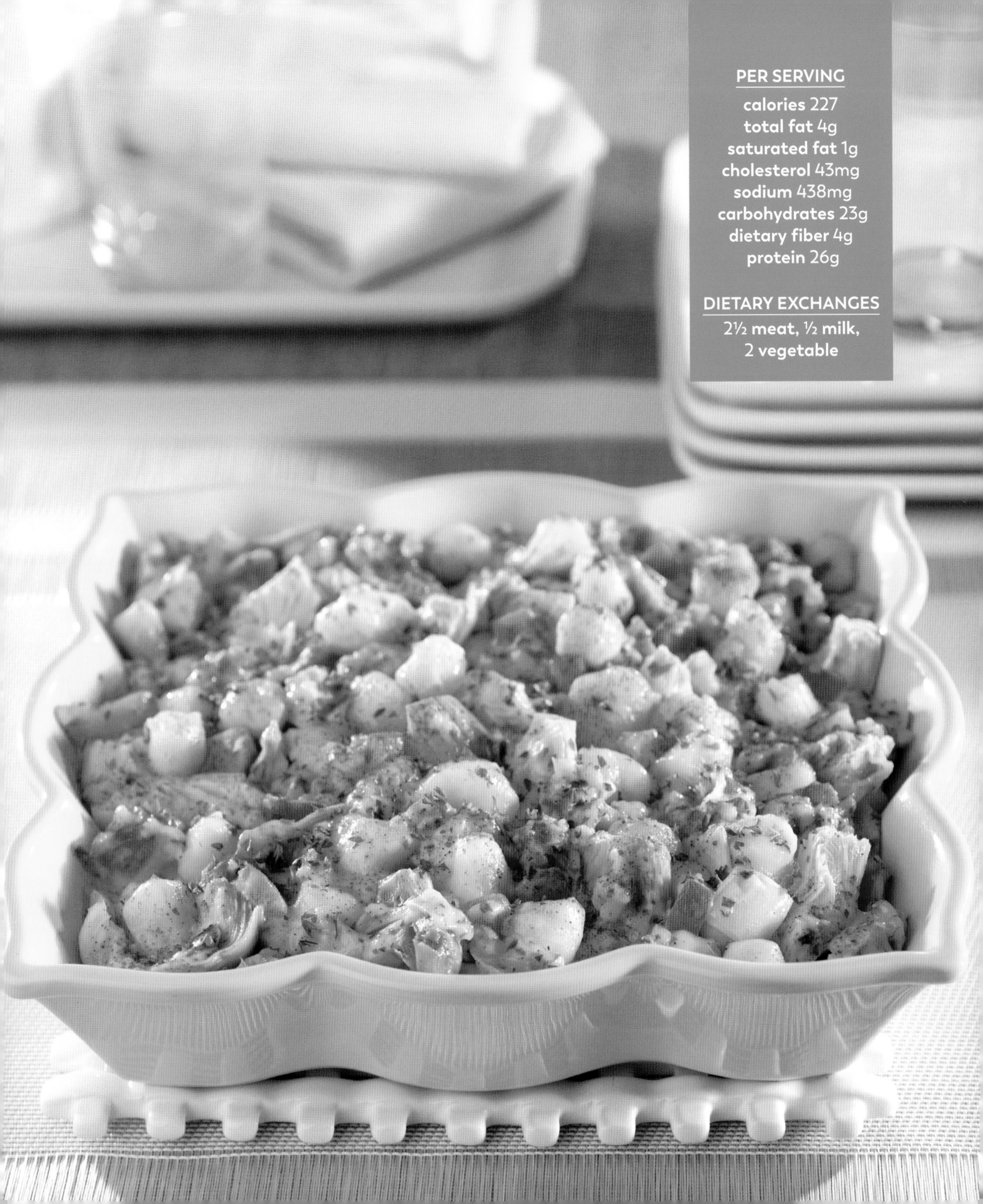

PER SERVING

calories 227
total fat 4g
saturated fat 1g
cholesterol 43mg
sodium 438mg
carbohydrates 23g
dietary fiber 4g
protein 26g

DIETARY EXCHANGES

2½ meat, ½ milk, 2 vegetable

Red Wine & Oregano Beef Kabobs

Makes 4 servings

¼ cup dry red wine

¼ cup finely chopped fresh parsley

2 tablespoons Worcestershire sauce

1 tablespoon reduced-sodium soy sauce

1 teaspoon dried oregano

3 cloves garlic, minced

½ teaspoon salt (optional)

½ teaspoon black pepper

¾ pound boneless beef top sirloin steak, cut into 16 (1-inch) pieces

16 whole mushrooms (about 8 ounces total)

1 medium red onion, cut in eighths and layers separated

1. Combine wine, parsley, Worcestershire sauce, soy sauce, oregano, garlic, salt, if desired, and pepper in small bowl; stir until well blended. Place steak, mushrooms and onion in large resealable food storage bag. Add wine mixture; seal bag and turn to coat. Marinate in refrigerator 1 hour, turning frequently.

2. Soak four (12-inch) or eight (6-inch) bamboo skewers in water for 20 minutes to prevent burning.

3. Preheat broiler. Alternate beef, mushrooms and 2 layers of onion on skewers.

4. Coat broiler rack with nonstick cooking spray. Arrange skewers on broiler rack; brush with marinade. Broil 4 to 6 inches from heat source 8 to 10 minutes, turning occasionally.

Tip: Pair the kabob with a side of whole grain brown rice, if your diet permits.

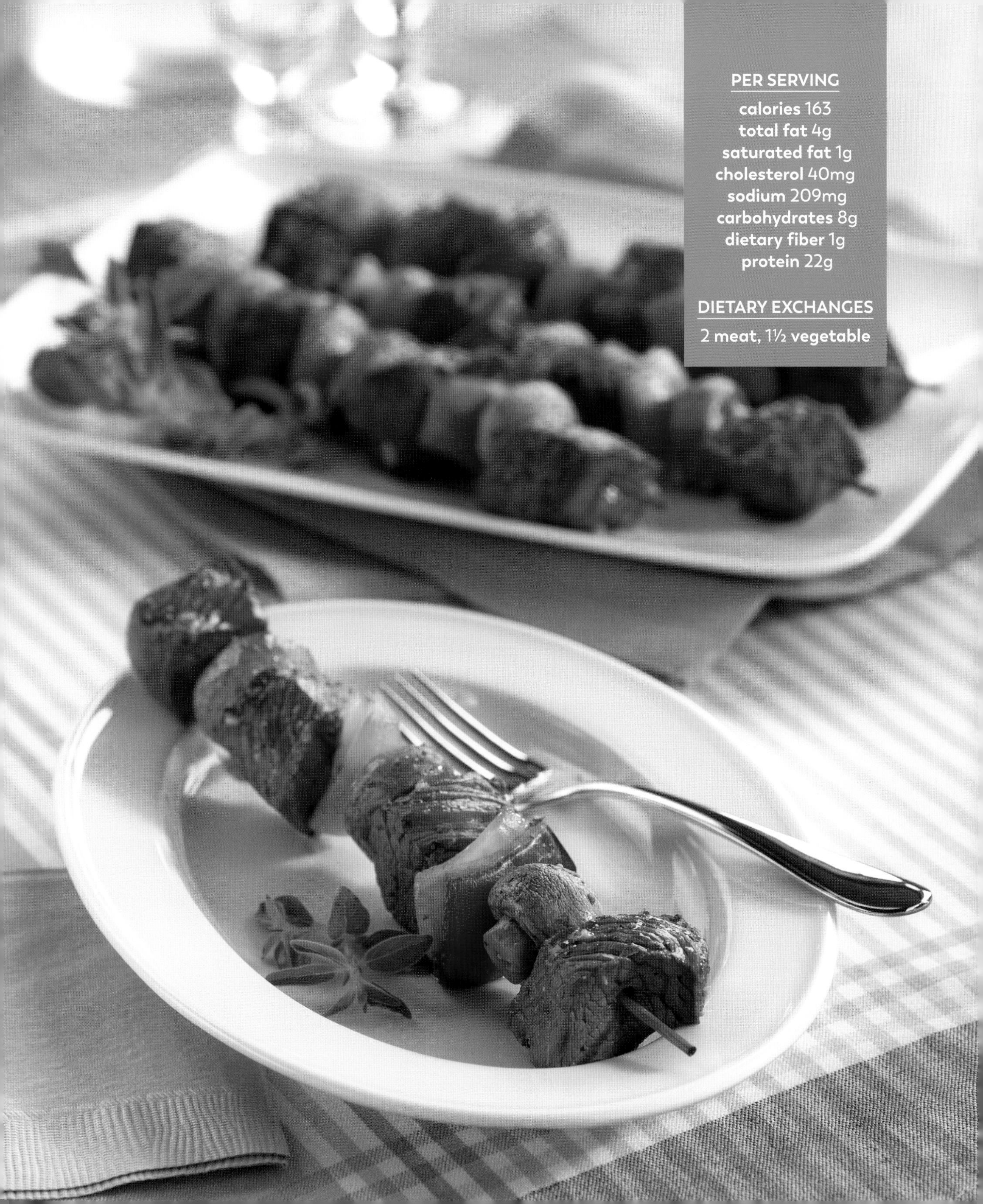

PER SERVING

calories 163
total fat 4g
saturated fat 1g
cholesterol 40mg
sodium 209mg
carbohydrates 8g
dietary fiber 1g
protein 22g

DIETARY EXCHANGES

2 meat, 1½ vegetable

Easy Make-at-Home Chinese Chicken

Makes 4 servings

3 tablespoons frozen orange juice concentrate, thawed

2 tablespoons water

2 tablespoons reduced-sodium soy sauce

¾ teaspoon cornstarch

¼ teaspoon garlic powder

2 carrots, sliced

1 package (12 ounces) frozen broccoli and cauliflower florets, thawed

2 teaspoons canola oil

¾ pound boneless skinless chicken breasts, cut into bite-sized pieces

1⅓ cups hot cooked rice

1. Combine orange juice concentrate, water, soy sauce, cornstarch and garlic powder in small bowl; stir until smooth.

2. Spray nonstick wok or large skillet with nonstick cooking spray. Add carrots; stir-fry over high heat 1 minute. Add broccoli and cauliflower; stir-fry 2 to 3 minutes or until vegetables are crisp-tender. Remove vegetables to medium bowl.

3. Add oil to wok; heat over medium-high heat. Add chicken; stir-fry 2 to 3 minutes or until cooked through. Push chicken up side of wok. Stir cornstarch mixture; add to wok. Bring to a boil. Return vegetables to wok; cook and stir until heated through. Serve over rice.

Tip: To cut carrots decoratively, use a citrus stripper or grapefruit spoon to cut 4 or 5 grooves into whole carrots, cutting lengthwise from stem end to tip. Then cut carrots crosswise into slices.

PER SERVING
calories 215
total fat 3g
saturated fat 1g
cholesterol 32mg
sodium 351mg
carbohydrates 29g
dietary fiber 4g
protein 18g

DIETARY EXCHANGES
1 bread/starch,
2 meat, 2 vegetable

Triple-Quick Shrimp and Pasta

Makes 4 servings

4 ounces uncooked whole grain rotini pasta

8 ounces small shrimp (with tails on), peeled

4 ounces asparagus spears, trimmed and broken into 2-inch pieces

1 cup grape tomatoes, quartered

½ cup light olive oil vinaigrette

2 cloves garlic, minced

2 teaspoons chopped fresh rosemary

¼ cup chopped fresh basil

¼ cup grated Parmesan cheese

1. Cook pasta according to package directions, omitting salt and fat. Add shrimp during last 4 minutes of cooking. Add asparagus during last 3 minutes of cooking; cook until shrimp are pink and opaque. Drain and return to saucepan.

2. Add tomatoes, vinaigrette, garlic and rosemary. Toss until well blended. Stir in basil and Parmesan cheese.

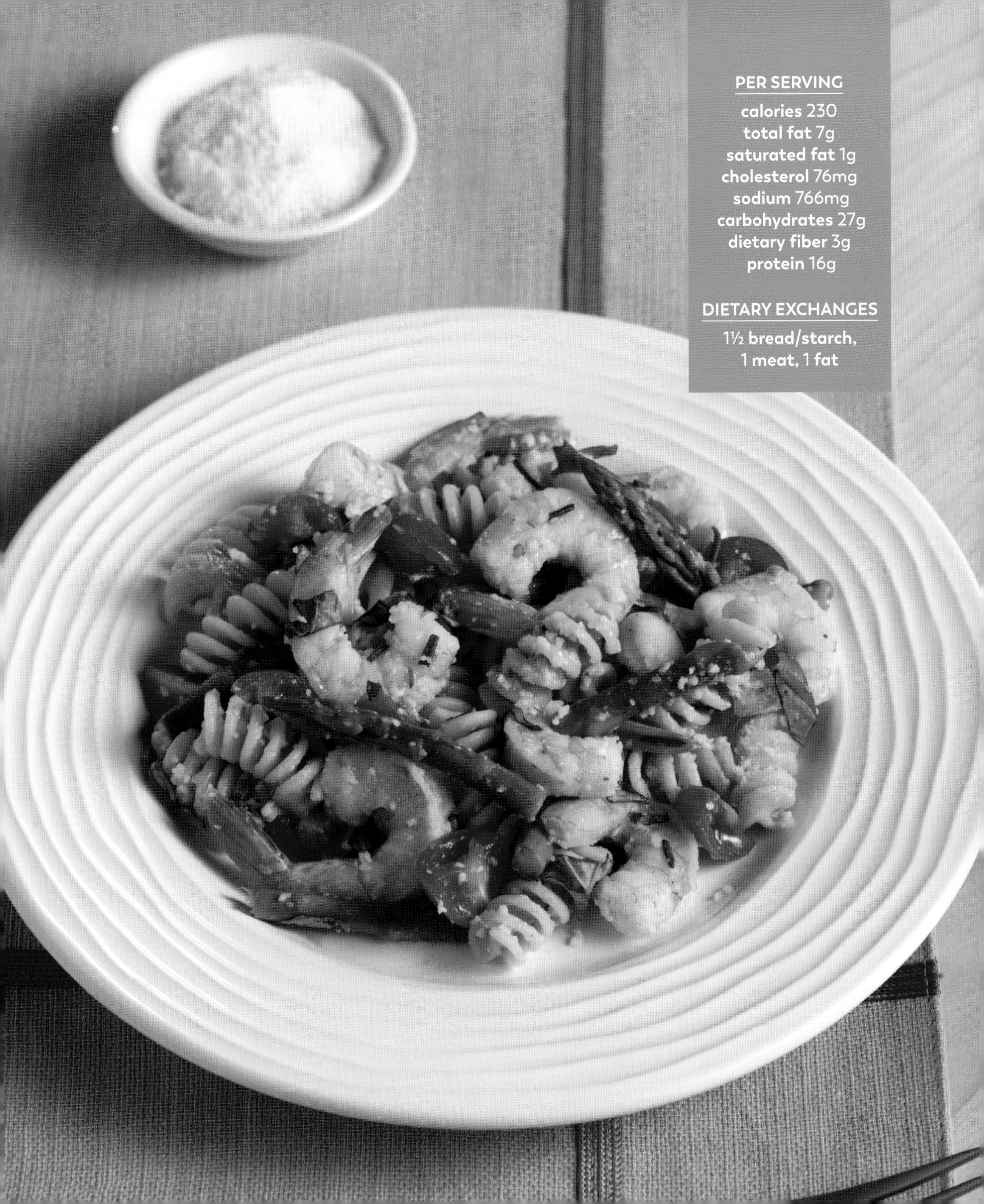

PER SERVING

calories 230
total fat 7g
saturated fat 1g
cholesterol 76mg
sodium 766mg
carbohydrates 27g
dietary fiber 3g
protein 16g

DIETARY EXCHANGES

1½ bread/starch, 1 meat, 1 fat

Provençal Lemon and Olive Chicken

Makes 8 servings

- 2 cups chopped onions
- 2 pounds skinless chicken thighs
- 1 medium lemon, thinly sliced and seeded
- ½ cup pitted green olives
- 1 tablespoon white vinegar *or* olive brine
- 2 teaspoons herbes de Provence
- 1 bay leaf
- ½ teaspoon salt
- ⅛ teaspoon black pepper
- 1 cup fat-free reduced-sodium chicken broth
- ½ cup minced fresh parsley
- Hot cooked rice (optional)

Slow Cooker Directions

1. Place onions in slow cooker. Arrange chicken thighs and lemon slices over onions. Add olives, vinegar, herbes de Provence, bay leaf, salt and pepper. Pour in broth.

2. Cover; cook on LOW 5 to 6 hours or on HIGH 3 to 3½ hours or until chicken is tender. Remove and discard bay leaf. Stir in parsley before serving.

3. Serve over rice, if desired.

PER SERVING
calories 180
total fat 7g
saturated fat 1.5g
cholesterol 105mg
sodium 380mg
carbohydrates 5g
dietary fiber 1g
protein 23g

DIETARY EXCHANGES
3 meat,
1 vegetable, ½ fat

Beef with Sweet Peppers and Eggplant

Makes 4 servings

1 ounce pine nuts (about
    3 tablespoons plus
    1 teaspoon) or slivered
    almonds (about ¼ cup)

¾ pound 95% lean ground beef

1 cup chopped yellow onion

⅓ medium eggplant (about
    8 ounces), peeled and cubed

1 cup chopped red bell pepper

½ cup water

1 can (8 ounces) tomato sauce
    with herbs

¾ teaspoon ground cinnamon

¼ teaspoon ground allspice

1 cup uncooked instant rice

½ teaspoon salt

1. Heat 12-inch nonstick skillet over medium-high heat until hot. Add pine nuts; cook, stirring constantly, 2 minutes or until pine nuts begin to lightly brown. Remove to plate; set aside.

2. Spray same skillet with nonstick cooking spray. Add beef and onions; cook and stir about 4 minutes or until beef is no longer pink. Add eggplant and bell pepper; coat lightly with cooking spray. Cook and stir 4 minutes or until eggplant is crisp-tender.

3. Add water; stir to blend. Add tomato sauce, cinnamon and allspice. Bring to a boil. Reduce heat. Cover tightly; simmer 10 minutes or until eggplant is tender and mixture has thickened slightly.

4. Meanwhile, cook rice according to package directions, omitting salt and fat.

5. Remove beef mixture from heat; stir salt and pine nuts into mixture. Cover tightly; let stand 5 minutes. Serve beef mixture over rice.

Easy Seafood Stir-Fry

Makes 4 servings

1 package (1 ounce) dried black Chinese mushrooms*

½ cup fat-free reduced-sodium chicken broth

2 tablespoons dry sherry

1 tablespoon reduced-sodium soy sauce

4½ teaspoons cornstarch

1 teaspoon vegetable oil, divided

8 ounces bay scallops or halved sea scallops

4 ounces medium raw shrimp, peeled and deveined

2 cloves garlic, minced

6 ounces (2 cups) fresh snow peas, cut diagonally into halves

2 cups hot cooked rice

¼ cup thinly sliced green onions

Or substitute 1½ cups sliced fresh mushrooms and omit step 1.

1. Place mushrooms in medium bowl; cover with warm water. Soak 20 to 40 minutes or until soft. Drain and squeeze out excess water. Cut off and discard stems; cut caps into thin slices.

2. Whisk broth, sherry, soy sauce and cornstarch in small bowl until smooth.

3. Heat ½ teaspoon oil in wok or large nonstick skillet over medium heat. Add scallops, shrimp and garlic; stir-fry 3 minutes or until seafood is opaque. Remove to large plate.

4. Heat remaining ½ teaspoon oil in wok. Add mushrooms and snow peas; stir-fry 3 minutes or until snow peas are crisp-tender. Stir broth mixture; add to wok. Stir-fry 2 minutes or until sauce boils and thickens.

5. Return seafood and any accumulated juices to wok; stir-fry until heated through. Serve with rice; sprinkle with green onions.

PER SERVING
calories 304
total fat 3g
saturated fat 1g
cholesterol 74mg
sodium 335mg
carbohydrates 42g
dietary fiber 3g
protein 25g

DIETARY EXCHANGES
2 bread/starch,
2 meat, 2 vegetable

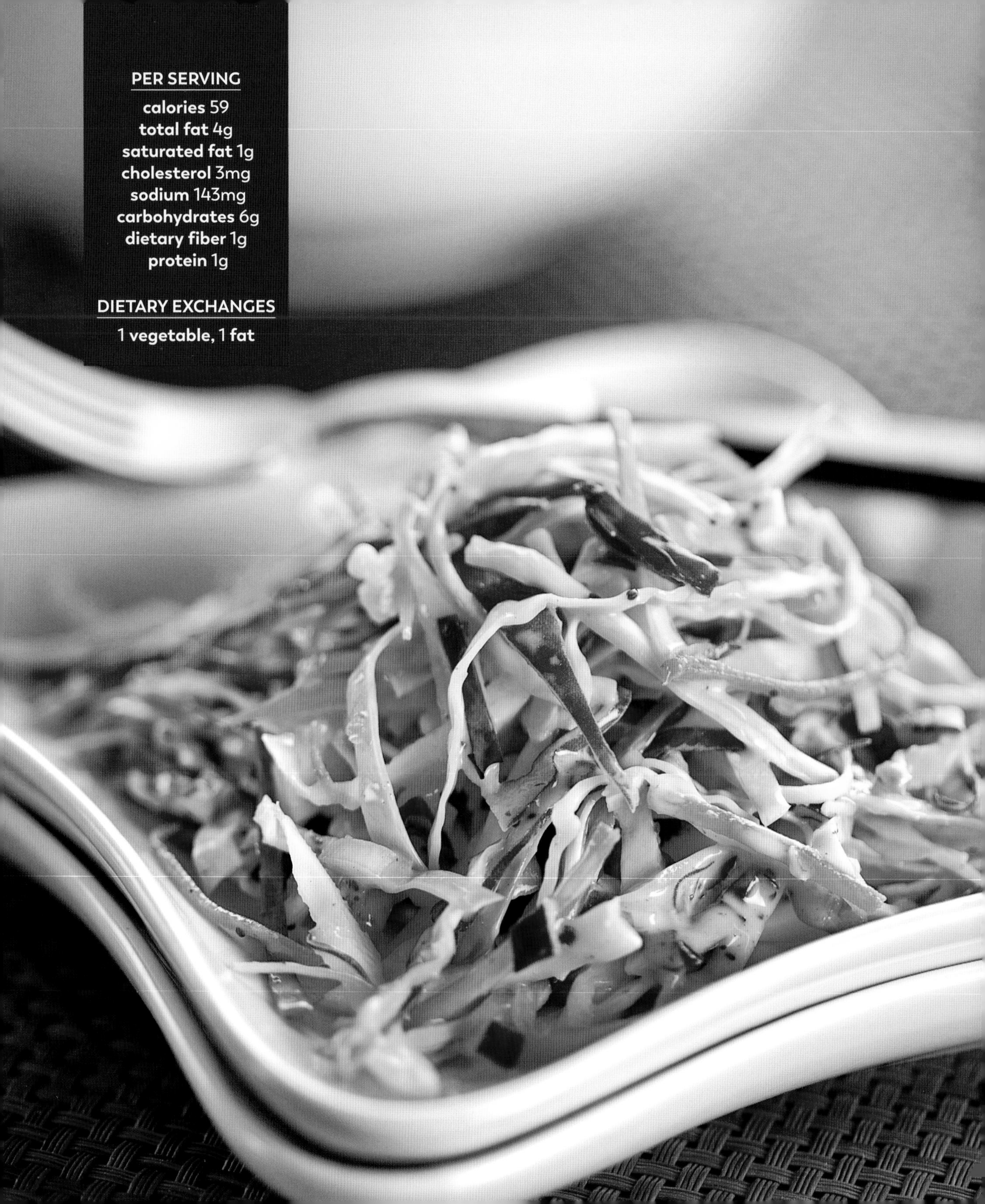

simple sides

Creamy Coleslaw

Makes 8 servings

- ½ cup light mayonnaise
- ½ cup low-fat buttermilk
- 2 teaspoons sugar
- 1 teaspoon celery seed
- 1 teaspoon fresh lime juice
- ½ teaspoon chili powder
- 3 cups shredded coleslaw mix
- 1 cup shredded carrots
- ¼ cup finely chopped red onion

Whisk mayonnaise, buttermilk, sugar, celery seed, lime juice and chili powder in large bowl until smooth and well blended. Add coleslaw mix, carrots and onion; toss to coat evenly. Cover and refrigerate at least 2 hours before serving.

Tofu "Fried" Rice

Makes 1 serving

- 2 ounces extra firm tofu
- ¼ cup finely chopped broccoli
- ¼ cup thawed frozen shelled edamame
- ⅓ cup cooked brown rice
- 1 tablespoon chopped green onion
- ½ teaspoon low-sodium soy sauce
- ⅛ teaspoon garlic powder
- ⅛ teaspoon sesame oil
- ⅛ teaspoon sriracha* or hot chili sauce (optional)

Sriracha is a Thai hot sauce that can be found in the ethnic section of major supermarkets or in Asian specialty markets.

Microwave Directions

1. Press tofu between paper towels to remove excess water. Cut into ½-inch cubes.

2. Combine tofu, broccoli and edamame in large microwavable mug; mix well. Microwave on HIGH 1 minute.

3. Stir in rice, green onion, soy sauce, garlic powder, oil and sriracha, if desired. Microwave 1 minute or until heated through. Stir well before serving.

PER SERVING
calories 210
total fat 7g
saturated fat 1g
cholesterol 0mg
sodium 118mg
carbohydrates 23g
dietary fiber 5g
protein 14g

DIETARY EXCHANGES
1 bread/starch,
1 meat, 1 vegetable,
1 fat

Sweet & Savory Sweet Potato Salad

Makes 6 servings

4 cups peeled chopped cooked sweet potatoes (about 4 to 6)

¾ cup chopped green onions

½ cup chopped fresh parsley

½ cup dried unsweetened cherries

¼ cup plus 2 tablespoons rice wine vinegar

2 tablespoons coarse ground mustard

1 tablespoon extra virgin olive oil

¾ teaspoon garlic powder

¼ teaspoon black pepper

⅛ teaspoon salt

1. Combine sweet potatoes, green onions, parsley and cherries in large bowl; gently mix.

2. Whisk vinegar, mustard, oil, garlic powder, pepper and salt in small bowl until well blended. Pour over sweet potato mixture; gently toss to coat. Serve immediately or cover and refrigerate until ready to serve.

PER SERVING
calories 161
total fat 3g
saturated fat 0g
cholesterol 0mg
sodium 116mg
carbohydrates 33g
dietary fiber 4g
protein 3g

DIETARY EXCHANGES
2 bread/starch, ½ fat

Couscous and Vegetable Risotto

Makes 4 servings

1   teaspoon olive oil

1   stalk celery, chopped

1   cup sliced mushrooms

1   medium yellow or orange bell pepper, cored, seeded and chopped

1   small onion, chopped

1   clove garlic, minced

¼   cup chopped fresh cranberries (optional)

¼   teaspoon dried crushed thyme

¼   teaspoon black pepper

⅔   cup uncooked pearl couscous

1½ to 1¾ cups reduced-sodium vegetable or chicken broth, divided

¼   teaspoon salt

1. Heat oil in large nonstick skillet over medium-high heat. Add celery, mushrooms, bell pepper, onion, garlic, cranberries, if desired, thyme and black pepper. Cook, stirring frequently 6 to 8 minutes or until celery is crisp-tender. Stir in couscous and cook 1 minute, stirring frequently.

2. Pour in ½ cup broth and scrape up browned bits in skillet. Reduce heat to medium-low. Stir in additional ½ cup broth. Cook, stirring occasionally, until broth is absorbed. Add another ½ cup broth. Cook, stirring occasionally. Taste. (Couscous should be tender, but not mushy, and the consistency should be creamy and thick.) If after 15 minutes couscous is still too firm, add remaining ¼ cup broth and repeat cooking and stirring. Stir in salt. Serve immediately.

Variation: Couscous and Vegetable Salad (pictured): Reserve ¾ cup Couscous and Vegetable Risotto; set aside. Combine 1 teaspoon Dijon mustard, 2 teaspoons olive oil, 1 tablespoon white wine vinegar, ¼ teaspoon black pepper, ⅛ teaspoon salt and 1 teaspoon chopped fresh chives in large bowl. Mix to combine. Add 8 ounces cut-up cooked asparagus, 1 cup cooked chopped chicken breast and reserved Risotto. Mix gently. Makes 2 servings.

PER SERVING
calories 165
total fat 2g
saturated fat 0g
cholesterol 0mg
sodium 366mg
carbohydrates 31g
dietary fiber 3g
protein 6g

DIETARY EXCHANGES
2 bread/starch, ½ fat

Mashed Potato Puffs

Makes 18 puffs (3 puffs per serving)

1 cup prepared mashed potatoes

½ cup finely chopped broccoli or spinach

2 egg whites

4 tablespoons shredded Parmesan cheese, divided

1. Preheat oven to 400°F. Spray 18 mini (1¾-inch) muffin cups with nonstick cooking spray.

2. Combine mashed potatoes, broccoli, egg whites and 2 tablespoons cheese in large bowl; mix well. Spoon evenly into prepared muffin cups. Sprinkle with remaining 2 tablespoons cheese.

3. Bake 20 to 23 minutes or until golden brown. To remove from pan, gently run knife around outer edges and lift out with fork. Serve warm.

PER SERVING
calories 63
total fat 2g
saturated fat 1g
cholesterol 2mg
sodium 99mg
carbohydrates 8g
dietary fiber 1g
protein 32g

DIETARY EXCHANGES
1 vegetable, ½ fat

Roasted Sweet Potato and Apple Salad

Makes 4 servings

2 large sweet potatoes, peeled and cubed

½ teaspoon salt, divided

¼ teaspoon black pepper

3 tablespoons low-calorie apple juice cocktail

1 tablespoon olive oil

1 tablespoon balsamic vinegar

1 tablespoon Dijon mustard

1 tablespoon honey

2 teaspoons snipped fresh chives

1 medium Gala apple, diced (about 1 cup)

½ cup finely chopped celery

¼ cup thinly sliced red onion

Lettuce leaves

1. Preheat oven to 450°F. Arrange sweet potatoes in single layer on baking sheet. Spray with nonstick cooking spray; season with ¼ teaspoon salt and pepper.

2. Roast 20 to 25 minutes or until potatoes are tender, stirring halfway through cooking time. Cool completely.

3. Meanwhile, whisk apple juice cocktail, oil, vinegar, mustard, honey, chives and remaining ¼ teaspoon salt in small bowl until smooth and well blended.

4. Combine sweet potatoes, apple, celery and onion in medium bowl. Drizzle with dressing; gently toss to coat. Arrange lettuce leaves on four serving plates. Top evenly with sweet potato mixture.

PER SERVING
calories 133
total fat 4g
saturated fat 1g
cholesterol 0mg
sodium 424mg
carbohydrates 26g
dietary fiber 3g
protein 1g

DIETARY EXCHANGES
1½ bread/starch,
½ fruit, ½ fat

Cold Peanut Noodle and Edamame Salad

Makes 4 servings

½ of an 8-ounce package brown rice pad thai noodles

3 tablespoons soy sauce

2 tablespoons dark sesame oil

2 tablespoons unseasoned rice vinegar

1 tablespoon sugar

1 tablespoon finely grated fresh ginger

1 tablespoon creamy peanut butter

1 tablespoon sriracha or hot chili sauce

2 teaspoons minced garlic

½ cup thawed frozen shelled edamame

¼ cup shredded carrots

¼ cup sliced green onions

Chopped peanuts (optional)

1. Prepare noodles according to package directions for pasta. Rinse under cold water; drain. Cut noodles into 3-inch lengths. Place in large bowl; set aside.

2. Whisk soy sauce, oil, vinegar, sugar, ginger, peanut butter, sriracha and garlic in small bowl until smooth and well blended.

3. Pour dressing over noodles; toss gently to coat. Stir in edamame and carrots. Cover and refrigerate at least 30 minutes before serving. Top with green onions and peanuts, if desired.

Note: Brown rice pad thai noodles can be found in the Asian section of the supermarket. Regular thin rice noodles or whole wheat spaghetti may be substituted.

Chopped Italian Salad

Makes 6 servings

10 cups chopped romaine lettuce

⅓ cup chopped red onion

20 slices low-fat turkey pepperoni, quartered (about 5 ounces)

1 can (2¼ ounces) sliced black olives, rinsed and drained

1 can (about 15 ounces) reduced-fat chickpeas, rinsed and drained

⅓ cup light balsamic vinaigrette dressing

⅓ cup shaved or grated reduced-fat Parmesan cheese

Combine lettuce, red onion, pepperoni, olives and chickpeas in large bowl. Add dressing; toss gently to coat. Sprinkle with cheese.

Sweet and Sour Broccoli Pasta Salad

Makes 6 servings

8 ounces uncooked pasta twists

2 cups broccoli florets

⅔ cup shredded carrots

1 medium Red or Golden Delicious apple, cored, seeded and chopped

⅓ cup plain nonfat yogurt

⅓ cup apple juice

3 tablespoons cider vinegar

1 tablespoon olive oil

1 tablespoon Dijon mustard

1 teaspoon honey

½ teaspoon dried thyme

Lettuce leaves

1. Cook pasta according to package directions, omitting salt. Add broccoli during the last 2 minutes of cooking; drain. Rinse under cold running water until pasta and broccoli are cool.

2. Combine pasta, broccoli, carrots and apple in medium bowl.

3. Whisk yogurt, apple juice, vinegar, oil, mustard, honey and thyme in small bowl until smooth and well blended. Pour over pasta mixture; toss to coat.

4. Line six plates with lettuce. Top evenly with pasta salad.

Carrot Raisin Salad with Citrus Dressing

Makes 8 servings

¾ cup light sour cream

¼ cup fat-free (skim) milk

1 tablespoon honey

1 tablespoon lime juice

1 tablespoon thawed frozen orange juice concentrate

Grated peel of 1 medium orange

¼ teaspoon salt

8 medium carrots, peeled and coarsely shredded (about 2 cups)

¼ cup raisins

⅓ cup chopped cashew nuts

1. Whisk sour cream, milk, honey, lime juice, orange juice concentrate, orange peel and salt in small bowl until smooth and well blended.

2. Combine carrots and raisins in large bowl. Add dressing; toss to coat. Cover and refrigerate 30 minutes. Gently toss before serving. Top with cashews.

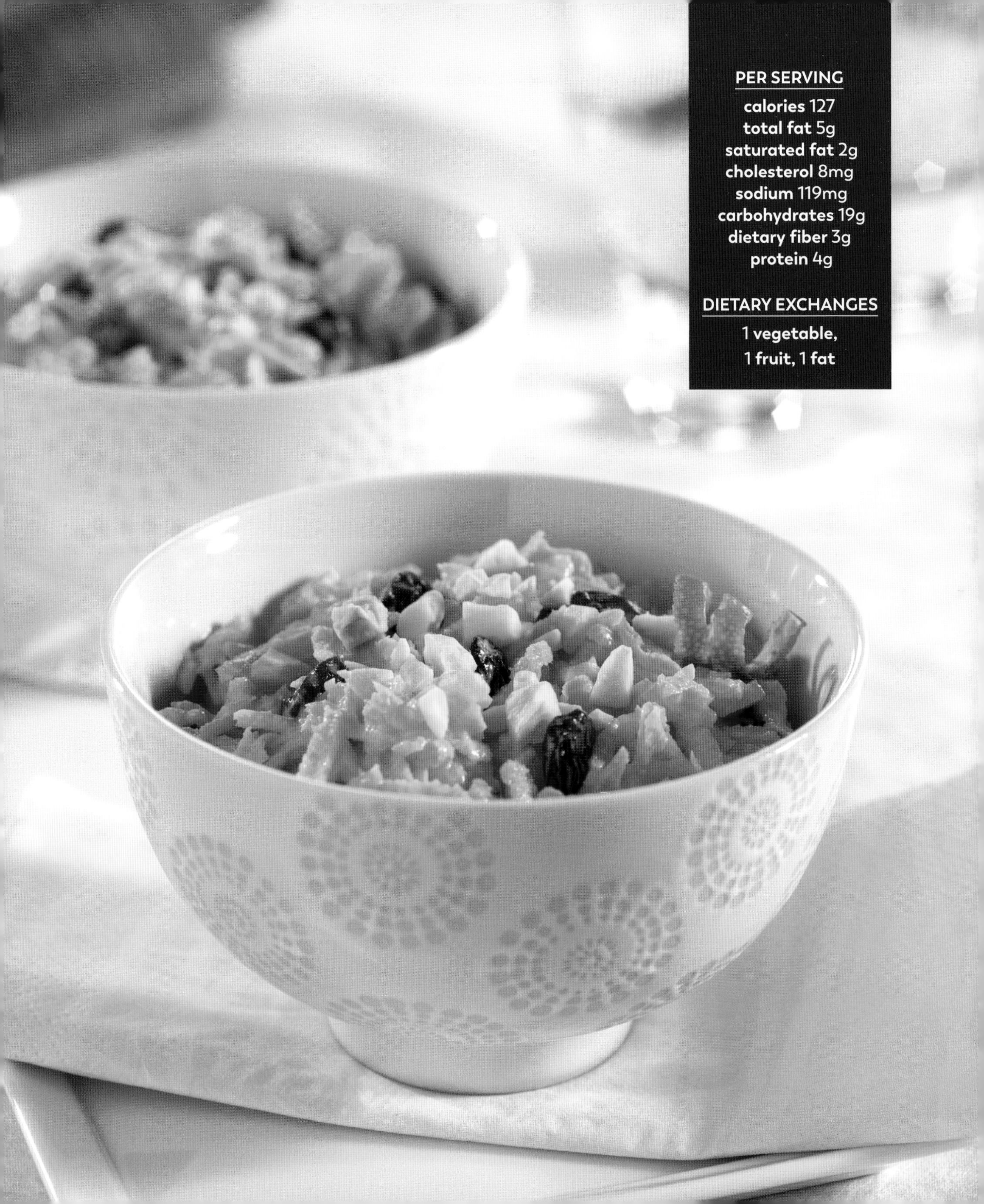

PER SERVING

calories 127
total fat 5g
saturated fat 2g
cholesterol 8mg
sodium 119mg
carbohydrates 19g
dietary fiber 3g
protein 4g

DIETARY EXCHANGES

1 vegetable, 1 fruit, 1 fat

Brown Rice with Chickpeas, Spinach and Feta

Makes 4 servings

½ cup diced celery

½ cup uncooked instant brown
    rice

1 can (about 15 ounces)
    reduced-sodium chickpeas,
    rinsed and drained

1 clove garlic, minced (optional)

1 package (10 ounces) frozen
    chopped spinach, thawed
    and drained

1 teaspoon Greek or Italian
    seasoning

¾ teaspoon vegetable broth

¼ teaspoon salt (optional)

⅛ teaspoon black pepper

2 cups water

1 tablespoon lemon juice

½ cup (2 ounces) crumbled
    fat-free feta cheese

1. Heat large skillet coated with nonstick cooking spray over medium-high heat. Add celery; cook, stirring occasionally, 4 minutes or until lightly glazed and brown in spots.

2. Add rice, chickpeas, garlic, if desired, spinach, Greek seasoning, broth, salt, if desired, pepper and water. Stir to combine. Cover and bring to a gentle boil. Reduce heat to low and boil gently 12 minutes or until rice is tender. Remove from heat; add lemon juice and feta. Mix gently with large spoon.

PER SERVING
calories 190
total fat 3g
saturated fat 0g
cholesterol 5mg
sodium 630mg
carbohydrates 29g
dietary fiber 7g
protein 16g

DIETARY EXCHANGES
1½ bread/starch,
1 meat, 1 vegetable

Heirloom Tomato Quinoa Salad

Makes 4 servings

1 cup uncooked quinoa

2 cups water

2 tablespoons olive oil

1 tablespoon lemon juice

1 clove garlic, minced

½ teaspoon salt

2 cups assorted heirloom grape tomatoes (red, yellow or a combination), halved

¼ cup crumbled fat-free feta cheese

¼ cup chopped fresh basil, plus additional basil leaves for garnish

1. Place quinoa in fine-mesh strainer; rinse well under cold running water. Bring 2 cups water to a boil in small saucepan; stir in quinoa. Reduce heat to low; cover and simmer 10 to 15 minutes or until quinoa is tender and water is absorbed.

2. Meanwhile, whisk oil, lemon juice, garlic and salt in large bowl until well blended. Gently stir in tomatoes and quinoa. Cover; refrigerate at least 30 minutes.

3. Stir in cheese just before serving. Top each serving with 1 tablespoon chopped basil. Garnish with additional basil leaves.

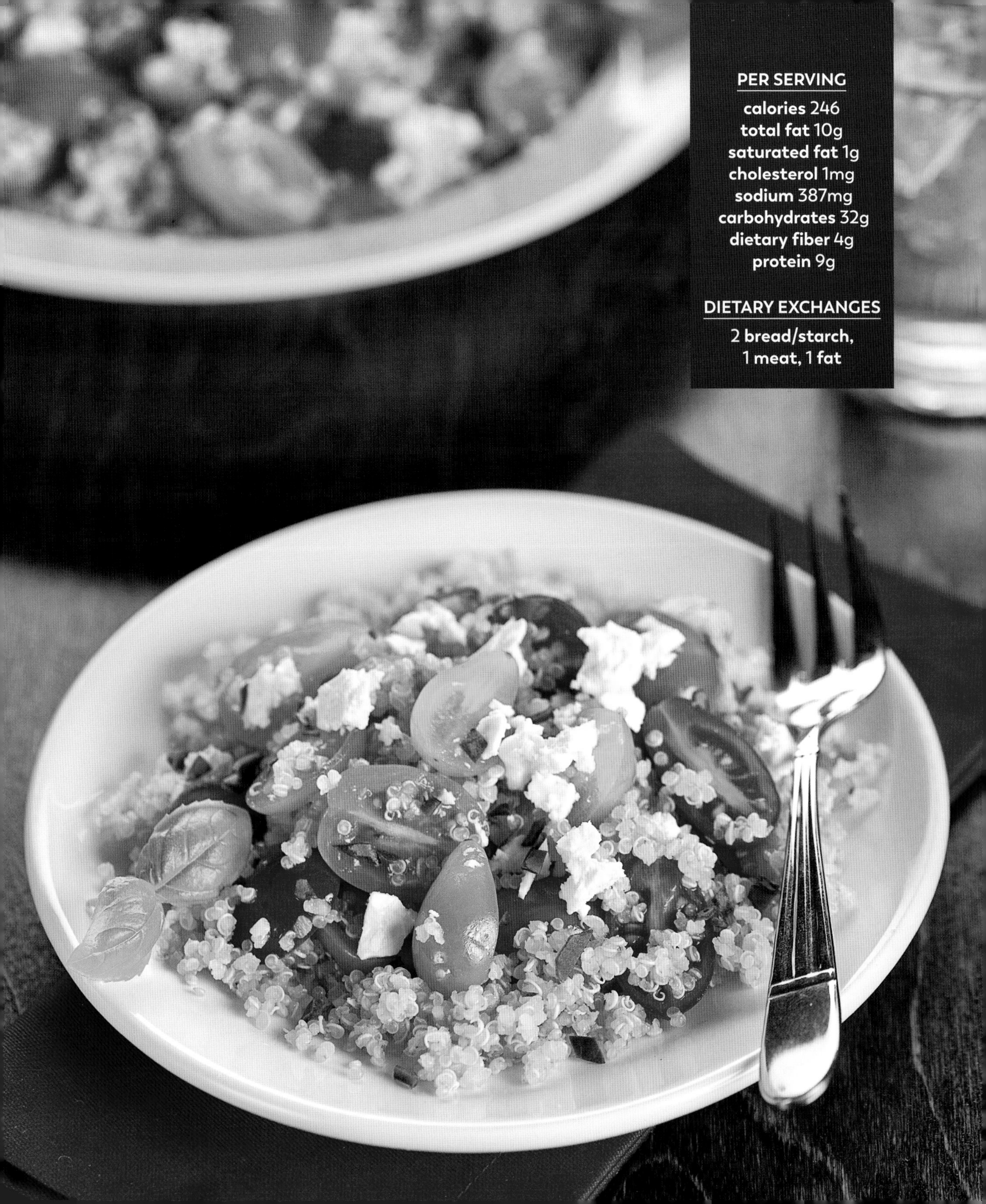

PER SERVING

calories 246
total fat 10g
saturated fat 1g
cholesterol 1mg
sodium 387mg
carbohydrates 32g
dietary fiber 4g
protein 9g

DIETARY EXCHANGES

2 **bread/starch,**
1 **meat,** 1 **fat**

Spicy Sesame Noodles

Makes 6 servings

- 6 ounces uncooked soba (buckwheat) noodles
- 2 teaspoons dark sesame oil
- 1 tablespoon sesame seeds
- ½ cup fat-free reduced-sodium chicken broth
- 1 tablespoon creamy peanut butter
- ½ cup thinly sliced green onions
- ½ cup minced red bell pepper
- 4 teaspoons reduced-sodium soy sauce
- 1½ teaspoons finely chopped seeded jalapeño pepper*
- 1 clove garlic, minced
- ¼ teaspoon red pepper flakes

*Jalapeño peppers can sting and irritate the skin, so wear rubber gloves when handling peppers and do not touch your eyes.

1. Cook noodles according to package directions. ***Do not overcook.*** Rinse noodles thoroughly with cold running water; drain. Place noodles in large bowl; toss with oil.

2. Cook sesame seeds in small skillet over medium heat about 3 minutes or until seeds begin to pop and turn golden brown, stirring frequently. Remove from skillet.

3. Whisk broth and peanut butter in medium bowl until blended. (Mixture may look curdled.) Stir in green onions, bell pepper, soy sauce, jalapeño pepper, garlic and red pepper flakes.

4. Pour mixture over noodles; toss to coat. Cover and let stand 30 minutes at room temperature or refrigerate up to 24 hours. Sprinkle with toasted sesame seeds before serving.

PER SERVING

calories 145
total fat 4g
saturated fat 1g
cholesterol 0mg
sodium 358mg
carbohydrates 24g
dietary fiber 1g
protein 6g

DIETARY EXCHANGES

1½ **bread/starch,**
½ **vegetable,** ½ **fat**

Marinated Vegetables

Makes 12 servings

¼ cup rice wine vinegar

3 tablespoons reduced-sodium soy sauce

2 tablespoons fresh lemon juice

1 tablespoon vegetable oil

1 clove garlic, minced

1 teaspoon minced fresh ginger

½ teaspoon sugar

2 cups broccoli florets

2 cups cauliflower florets

2 cups diagonally sliced carrots (½-inch pieces)

8 ounces whole fresh mushrooms

1 large red bell pepper, cut into 1-inch pieces

Lettuce leaves

1. Combine vinegar, soy sauce, lemon juice, oil, garlic, ginger and sugar in large bowl. Set aside.

2. To blanch broccoli, cauliflower and carrots, cook 1 minute in enough salted boiling water to cover. Remove and plunge into cold water, then drain immediately. Add to oil mixture in bowl while still warm; toss to coat. Cool to room temperature.

3. Add mushrooms and bell pepper to vegetables in bowl; toss to coat. Cover and marinate in refrigerator at least 4 hours or up to 24 hours. Drain vegetables, reserving marinade.

4. Arrange vegetables on lettuce-lined platter. Serve chilled or at room temperature with toothpicks. Serve remaining marinade in small cup for dipping, if desired.

PER SERVING
calories 37
total fat 1g
saturated fat 1g
cholesterol 0mg
sodium 146mg
carbohydrates 6g
dietary fiber 2g
protein 2g

DIETARY EXCHANGES
1 vegetable

Toasted Peanut Couscous Salad

Makes 4 servings

½ cup water

¼ cup uncooked couscous

½ cup finely chopped red onion

½ cup finely chopped green bell pepper

1 ounce unsalted dry-roasted peanuts

1 tablespoon reduced-sodium soy sauce

2 teaspoons cider vinegar

1½ teaspoons sesame oil

½ teaspoon grated fresh ginger

1 packet sugar substitute*

¼ teaspoon salt

⅛ teaspoon red pepper flakes

This recipe was tested using sucralose-based sugar substitute.

1. Bring water to a boil in small saucepan over high heat. Remove from heat; stir in couscous. Cover tightly and let stand 5 minutes or until water is absorbed. Place in medium bowl; cool slightly. Stir in onion and bell pepper.

2. Heat small nonstick skillet over medium-high heat until hot. Add peanuts; cook 2 to 3 minutes or until beginning to turn golden, stirring frequently. Add to couscous.

3. Whisk soy sauce, vinegar, oil, ginger, sugar substitute, salt and red pepper flakes in small bowl. Add to couscous; stir until well blended.

PER SERVING

calories 115
total fat 5g
saturated fat 1g
cholesterol 0mg
sodium 298mg
carbohydrates 14g
dietary fiber 2g
protein 4g

DIETARY EXCHANGES

1 bread/starch, 1 fat

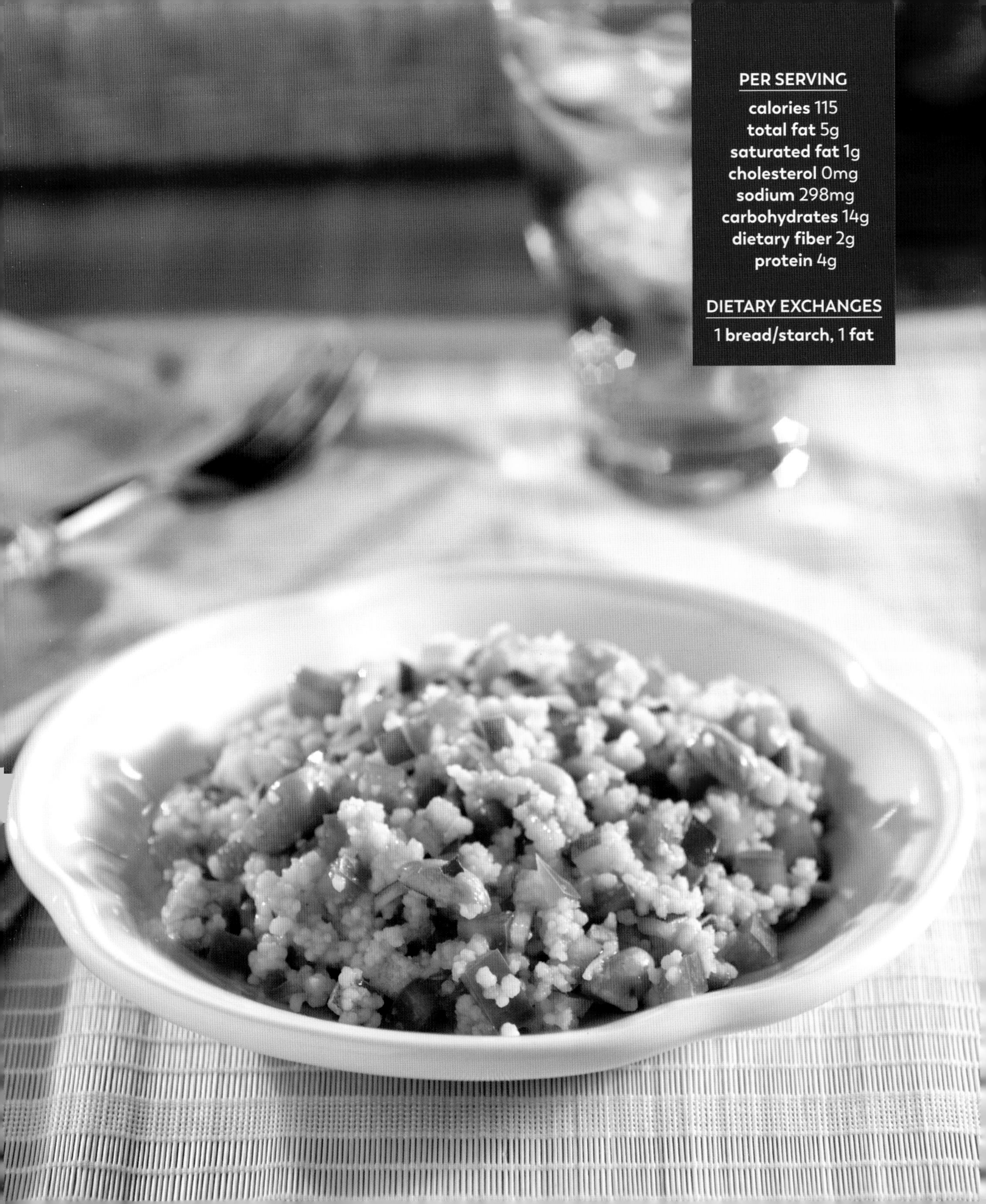

PER SERVING

calories 38
total fat 2g
saturated fat 0g
cholesterol 0mg
sodium 101mg
carbohydrates 4g
dietary fiber 1g
protein 1g

DIETARY EXCHANGES

1 vegetable, ½ fat

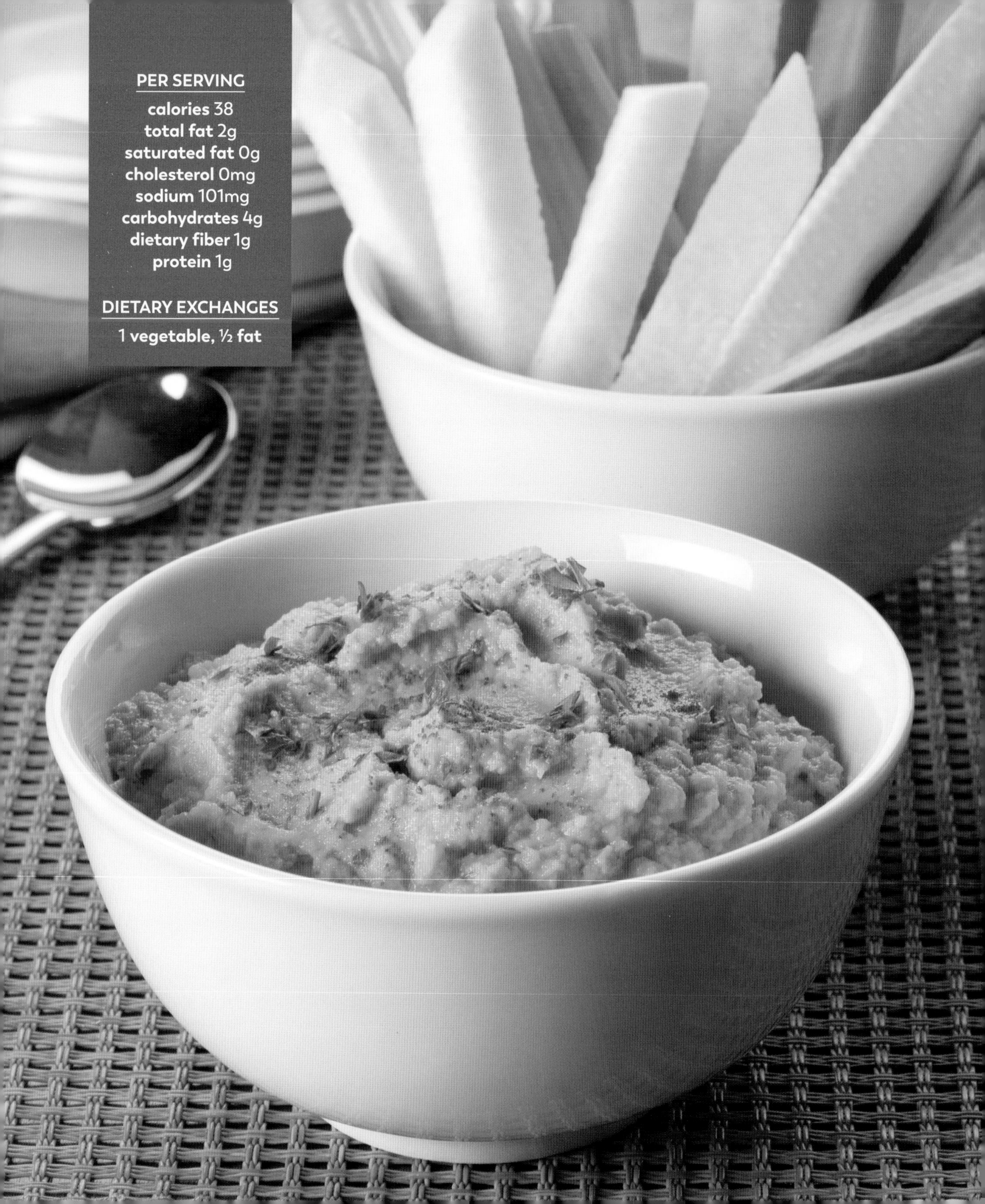

satisfying snacks

Savory Pumpkin Hummus

Makes 1½ cups (about 12 servings)

1   **can (15 ounces) solid-pack pumpkin**

3   **tablespoons chopped fresh parsley, plus additional for garnish**

3   **tablespoons tahini**

3   **tablespoons lemon juice**

3   **cloves garlic**

1   **teaspoon ground cumin**

½   **teaspoon salt**

⅛   **teaspoon black pepper**

⅛   **teaspoon ground red pepper, plus additional for garnish**

    Assorted vegetable sticks

1. Combine pumpkin, 3 tablespoons parsley, tahini, lemon juice, garlic, cumin, salt, black pepper and ⅛ teaspoon ground red pepper in food processor or blender; process until smooth. Cover and refrigerate at least 2 hours to allow flavors to develop.

2. Sprinkle with additional ground red pepper, if desired. Garnish with additional parsley. Serve with assorted vegetable sticks.

Southwest Snack Mix

Makes about 12 servings

4 cups unsweetened corn cereal squares

2 cups unsalted pretzels

½ cup unsalted pumpkin or squash seeds

1½ teaspoons chili powder

1 teaspoon minced fresh cilantro or parsley

½ teaspoon garlic powder

½ teaspoon onion powder

1 egg white

2 tablespoons olive oil

2 tablespoons lime juice

1. Preheat oven to 300°F. Spray baking sheet with nonstick cooking spray.

2. Combine cereal, pretzels and pumpkin seeds in large bowl. Combine chili powder, cilantro, garlic powder and onion powder in small bowl.

3. Whisk egg white, oil and lime juice in separate small bowl until well blended. Pour over cereal mixture; toss to coat. Add seasoning mixture; mix lightly to coat evenly. Transfer to prepared baking sheet.

4. Bake 45 minutes, stirring every 15 minutes. Cool completely. Store in airtight container.

Variation: Substitute ½ cup unsalted peanuts for pumpkin seeds.

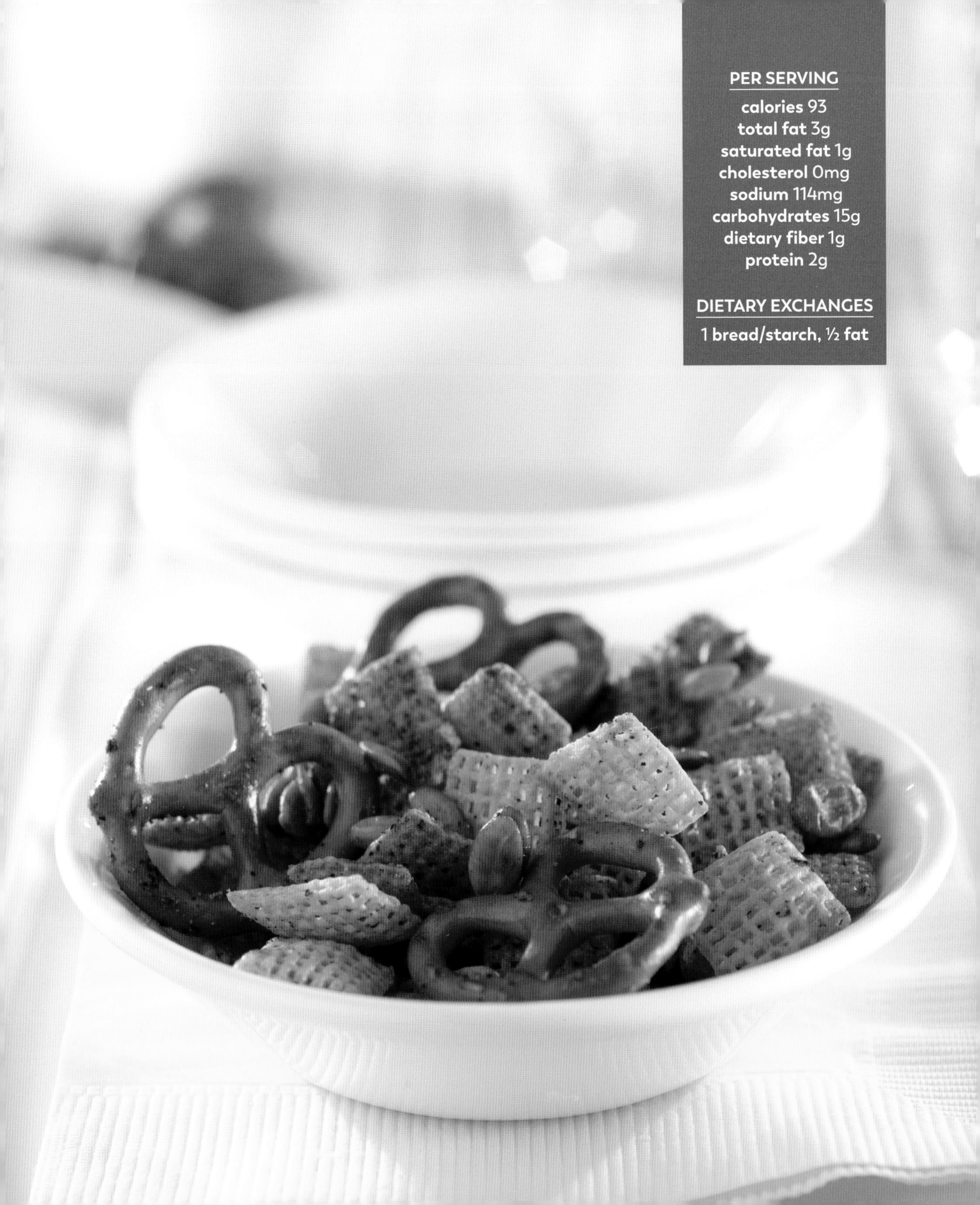

PER SERVING

calories 93
total fat 3g
saturated fat 1g
cholesterol 0mg
sodium 114mg
carbohydrates 15g
dietary fiber 1g
protein 2g

DIETARY EXCHANGES

1 bread/starch, ½ fat

Pear-Topped Grahams

Makes 4 servings

¼ cup low-fat cream cheese

4 whole cinnamon graham crackers

4 teaspoons raspberry fruit spread

1 pear, halved, cored and cut into 16 slices

1. Spread 1 tablespoon cream cheese evenly over each whole cracker. Spoon 1 teaspoon fruit spread on top.

2. Arrange 4 pear slices overlapping slightly on top of each cracker. Serve immediately.

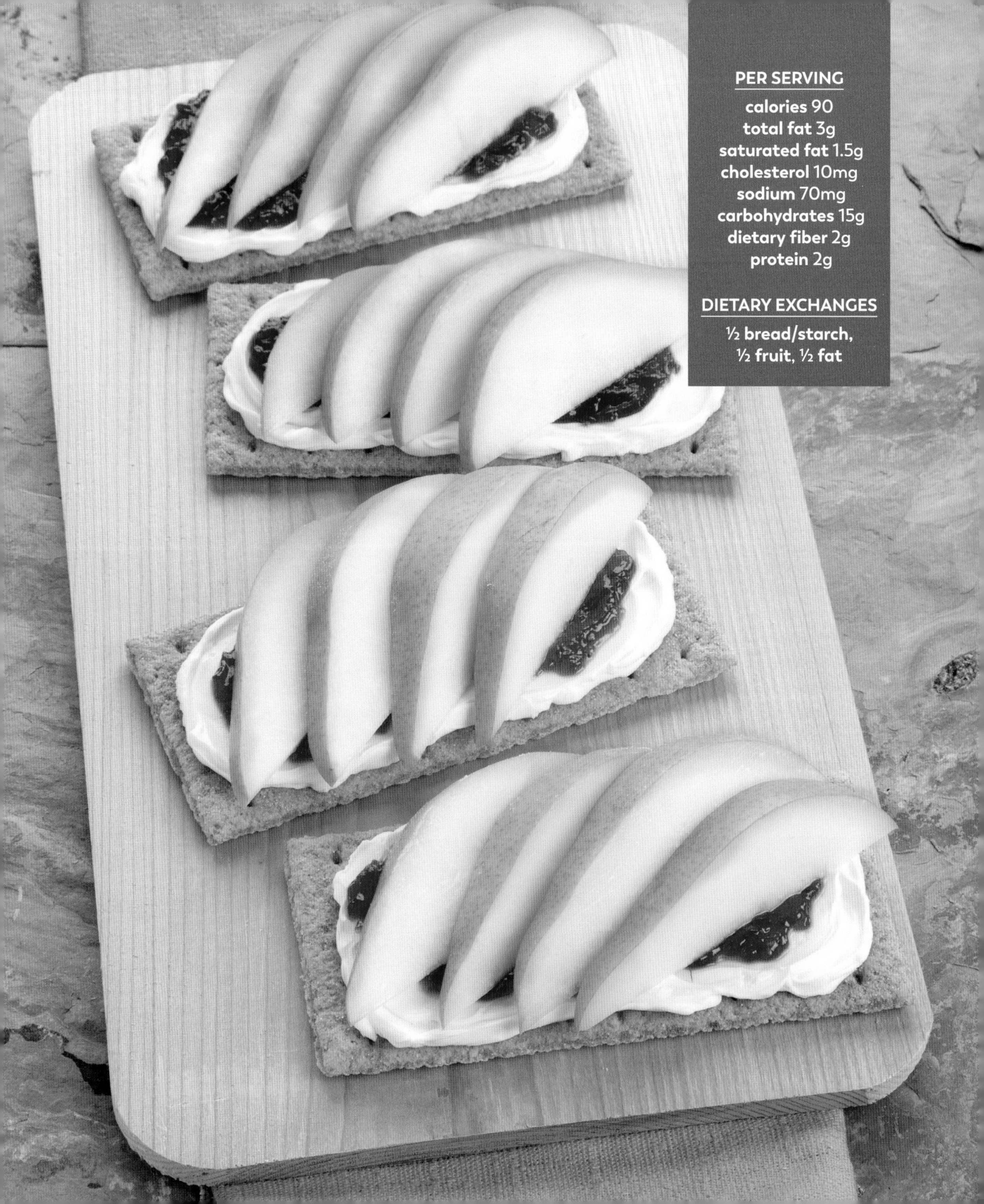

PB Banana Muffins

Makes 18 muffins

¾ cup all-purpose flour

¾ cup whole wheat flour

1 teaspoon baking soda

½ teaspoon salt

¾ cup reduced-fat creamy peanut butter

2 ripe bananas, mashed (about 1 cup)

½ cup packed brown sugar

½ cup plain nonfat yogurt

1 egg

¼ cup honey

¼ cup vegetable oil

1 teaspoon vanilla

1. Preheat oven to 375°F. Line 18 standard (2½-inch) muffin cups with paper baking cups or spray with nonstick cooking spray.

2. Combine all-purpose flour, whole wheat flour, baking soda and salt in medium bowl; mix well. Beat peanut butter, bananas, brown sugar, yogurt, egg, honey, oil and vanilla in large bowl with electric mixer at medium speed until smooth and well blended. Add flour mixture; beat on low speed just until combined. Spoon batter evenly into prepared muffin cups.

3. Bake 15 to 18 minutes or until toothpick inserted into centers comes out clean. Cool in pans 5 minutes. Remove to wire racks; cool completely.

PER SERVING
calories 184
total fat 8g
saturated fat 1g
cholesterol 10mg
sodium 223mg
carbohydrates 25g
dietary fiber 2g
protein 4g

DIETARY EXCHANGES
1½ bread/starch,
1½ fat

Garlic-Parmesan Popcorn

Makes 12 cups popcorn (2 cups per serving)

1 tablespoon olive oil

1 clove garlic, finely minced

1 tablespoon light butter-and-oil spread, melted

12 cups plain popped popcorn

⅓ cup finely grated Parmesan cheese

½ teaspoon dried basil

½ teaspoon dried oregano

1. Stir oil and garlic into spread in small bowl until well blended. Pour over popcorn in large bowl; toss to coat.

2. Sprinkle with cheese, basil and oregano.

Tip: One regular-size microwavable package of popcorn yields about 10 to 12 cups of popped popcorn.

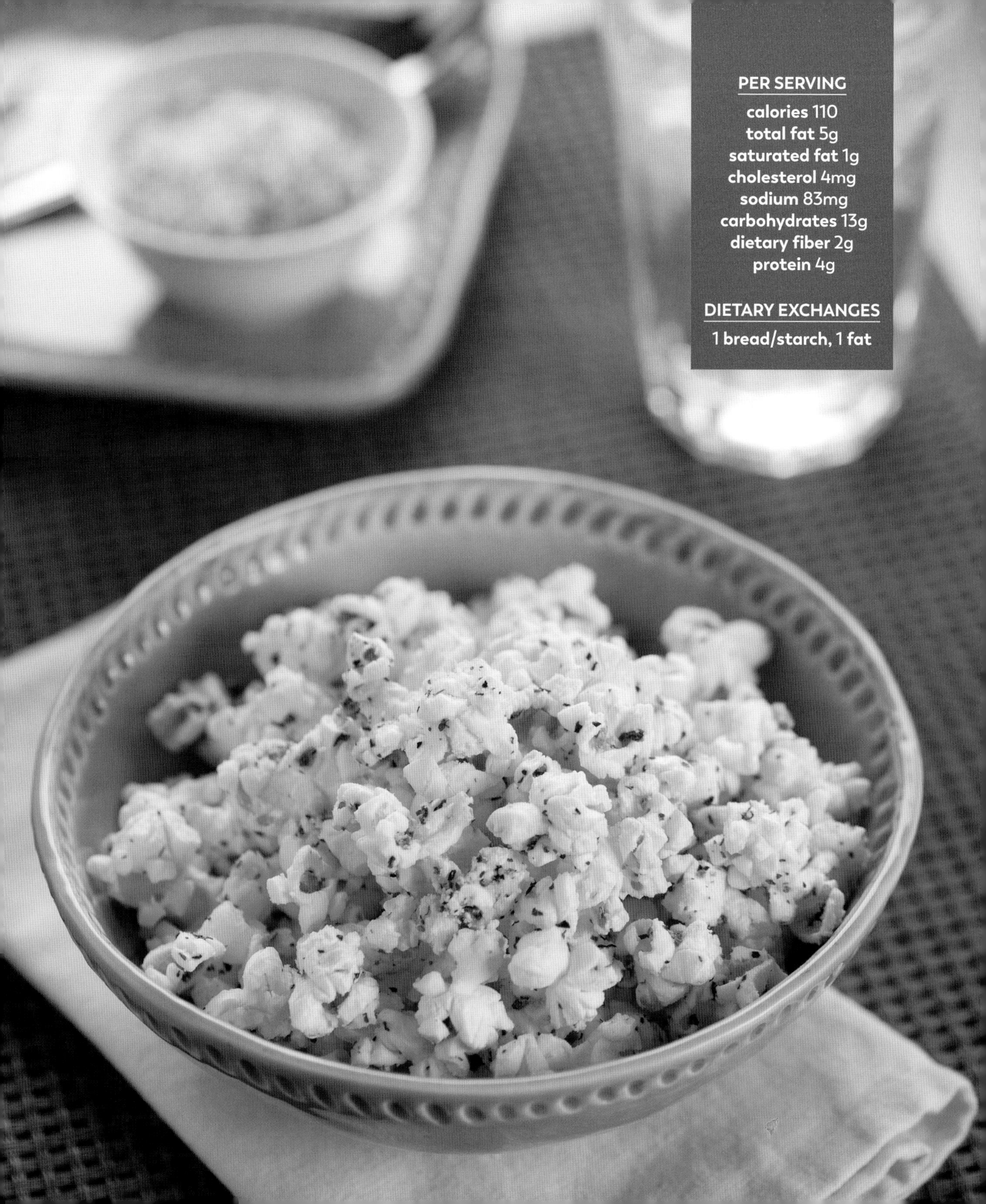

PER SERVING

calories 110
total fat 5g
saturated fat 1g
cholesterol 4mg
sodium 83mg
carbohydrates 13g
dietary fiber 2g
protein 4g

DIETARY EXCHANGES

1 bread/starch, 1 fat

Gingerbread Pineapple Muffins

Makes 24 servings

1 can (8 ounces) crushed pineapple in juice, undrained

1 package (14½ ounces) gingerbread cake and cookie mix

¾ cup lukewarm water

1 egg

2 teaspoons canola oil

¼ cup chopped walnuts (optional)

Powdered sugar (optional)

1. Preheat oven to 350°F. Spray mini muffin pan with nonstick cooking spray.

2. Place pineapple with juice in fine sieve over medium bowl; drain well, pressing pineapple to release juices. Retain juice.

3. Combine gingerbread mix, water, pineapple juice, egg and oil in large bowl; whisk 2 full minutes, scraping side often. Stir in walnuts, if desired.

4. Spoon batter into prepared muffin cups. Top each with equal amount of pineapple. Bake 13 to 16 minutes or until toothpick inserted into centers comes out clean.

5. Remove to cooling rack; cool completely. Sprinkle lightly with powdered sugar, if desired.

Note: After these muffins are completely cooled, they can be stored in an airtight container for up to 2 days.

PER SERVING
calories 87
total fat 3g
saturated fat 1g
cholesterol 9mg
sodium 116mg
carbohydrates 14g
dietary fiber 1g
protein 1g

DIETARY EXCHANGES
1 bread/starch

Fast Guacamole and "Chips"

Makes 8 servings

2 ripe avocados

½ cup chunky salsa

¼ teaspoon hot pepper sauce (optional)

½ seedless cucumber, sliced into ⅛-inch-thick rounds

1. Cut avocados in half; remove and discard pits. Scoop flesh into medium bowl; mash with fork.

2. Add salsa and hot pepper sauce, if desired; mix well.

3. Transfer guacamole to serving bowl. Serve with cucumber "chips."

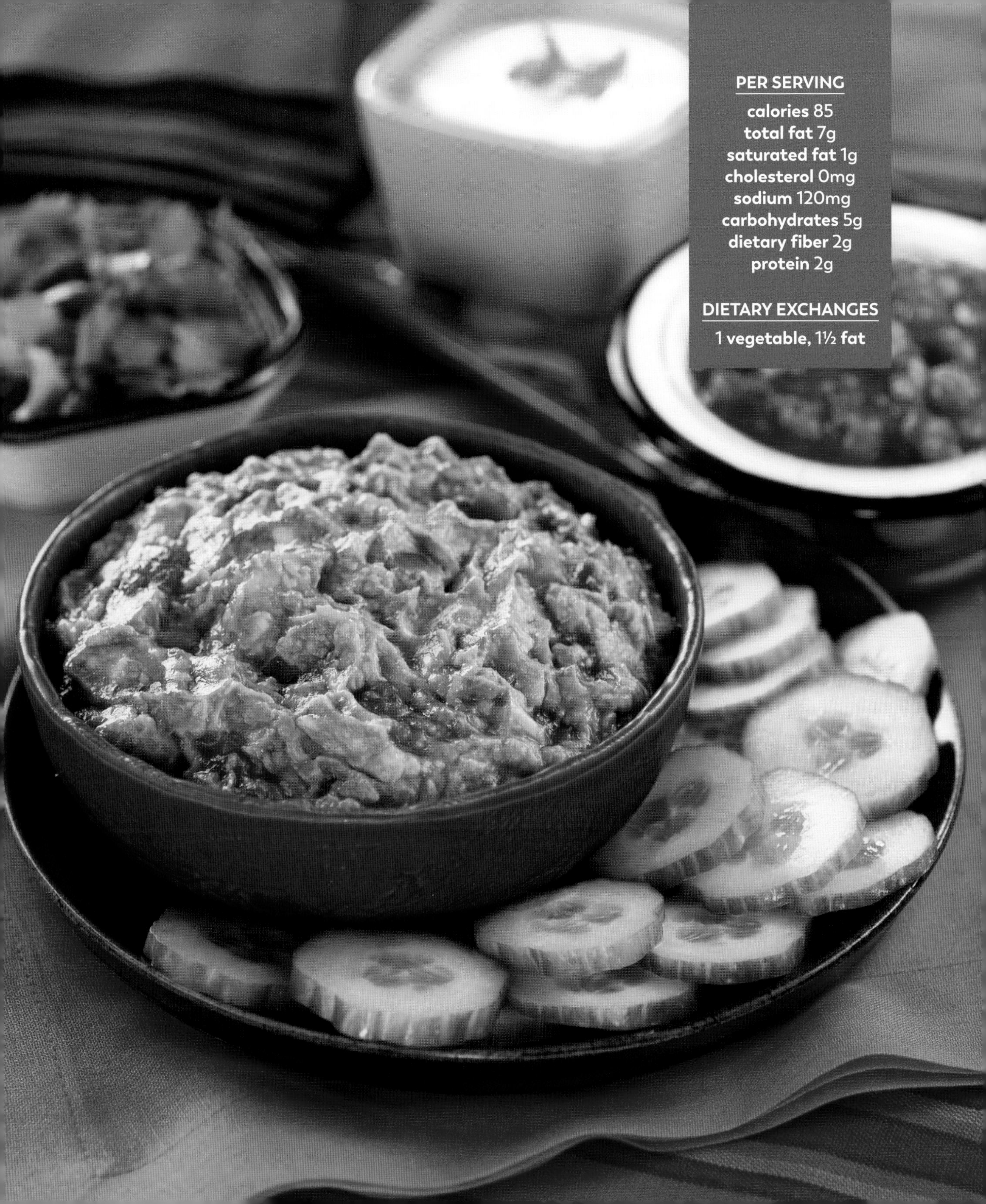

PER SERVING

calories 85
total fat 7g
saturated fat 1g
cholesterol 0mg
sodium 120mg
carbohydrates 5g
dietary fiber 2g
protein 2g

DIETARY EXCHANGES

1 vegetable, 1½ fat

Banana-Pecan Bread

Makes 1 loaf (about 16 servings)

3 large ripe bananas, mashed (about 1⅓ cups)

½ cup packed dark brown sugar

¼ cup granulated sugar

2 eggs, lightly beaten

¼ cup fat-free (skim) milk

¼ cup canola oil

2 cups reduced-fat biscuit baking mix

1 teaspoon ground cinnamon

½ cup golden raisins

½ cup chopped pecans

1. Preheat oven to 350°F. Spray 9×5-inch loaf pan with nonstick cooking spray; dust with flour.

2. Combine bananas, brown sugar, granulated sugar, eggs, milk and oil in large bowl; mix well. Stir in baking mix and cinnamon until well blended. Fold in raisins and pecans. Pour batter into prepared pan.

3. Bake 45 to 50 minutes or until top is golden brown and toothpick inserted into center comes out clean. Cool in pan on wire rack 20 minutes. Remove to wire rack; serve warm or cool completely.

PER SERVING
calories 183
total fat 8g
saturated fat 1g
cholesterol 23mg
sodium 176mg
carbohydrates 28g
dietary fiber 1g
protein 3g

DIETARY EXCHANGES
2 bread/starch, 1 fat

Fruit & Nut Quinoa

Makes 6 servings

- 1 cup uncooked quinoa
- 2 cups water
- 2 tablespoons finely grated orange peel, plus additional for garnish
- ¼ cup fresh orange juice
- 2 teaspoons olive oil
- ½ teaspoon salt
- ¼ teaspoon ground cinnamon
- ⅓ cup dried cranberries
- ⅓ cup toasted pistachio nuts*

*To toast pistachios, spread in single layer in heavy skillet. Cook and stir over medium heat 1 to 2 minutes or until nuts are lightly browned.

1. Place quinoa in fine-mesh strainer; rinse well under cold running water.

2. Bring 2 cups water to a boil in medium saucepan over high heat; stir in quinoa. Reduce heat to low; cover and simmer 10 to 15 minutes or until quinoa is tender and water is absorbed. Stir in 2 tablespoons orange peel.

3. Whisk orange juice, oil, salt and cinnamon in small bowl. Pour over quinoa; gently toss to coat. Fold in cranberries and pistachios. Serve warm or at room temperature. Garnish with additional orange peel.

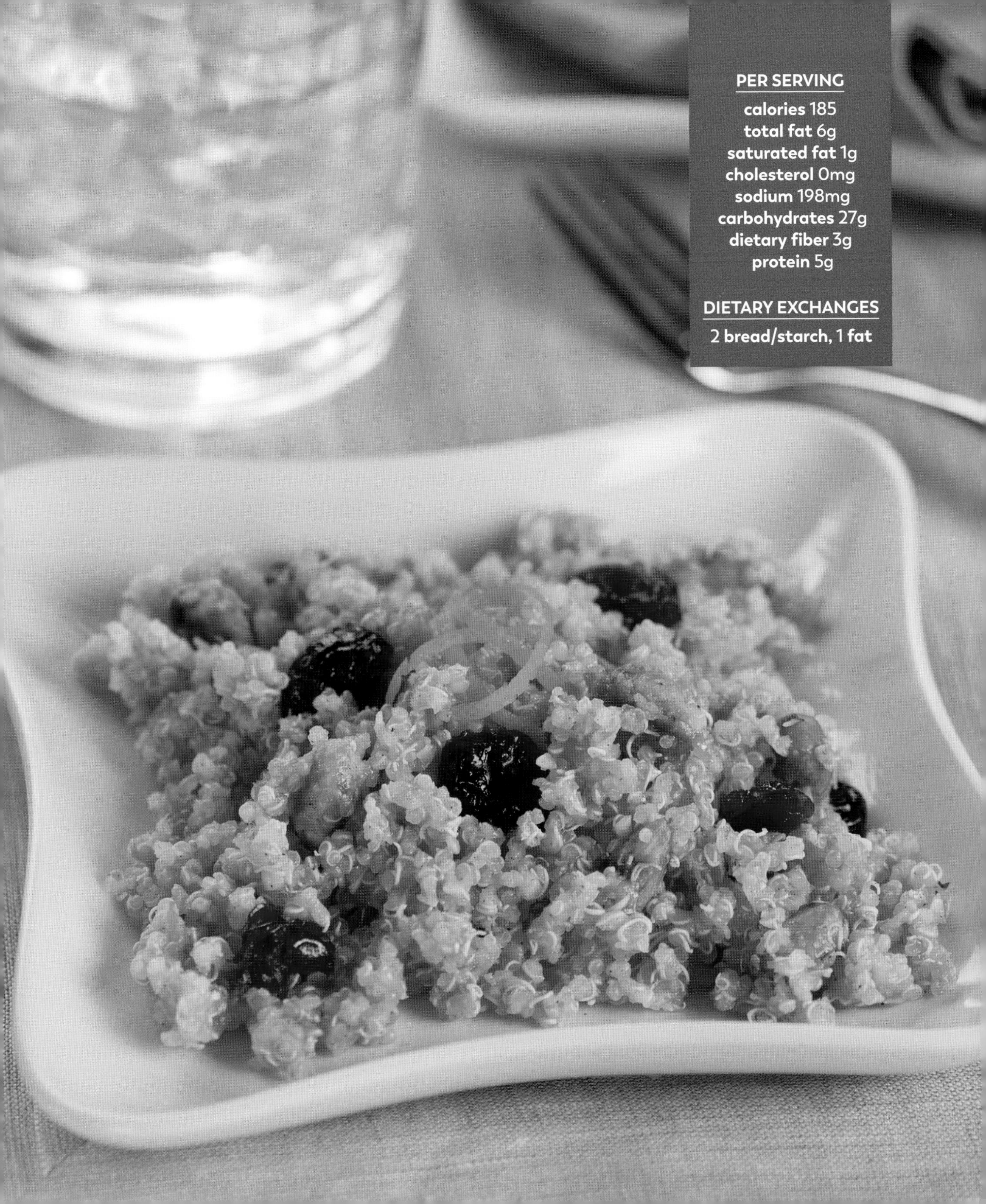

PER SERVING

calories 185
total fat 6g
saturated fat 1g
cholesterol 0mg
sodium 198mg
carbohydrates 27g
dietary fiber 3g
protein 5g

DIETARY EXCHANGES

2 bread/starch, 1 fat

PER SERVING

calories 205
total fat 3g
saturated fat 1g
cholesterol 0mg
sodium 335mg
carbohydrates 42g
dietary fiber 4g
protein 4g

DIETARY EXCHANGES

2 bread/starch, 1 fruit

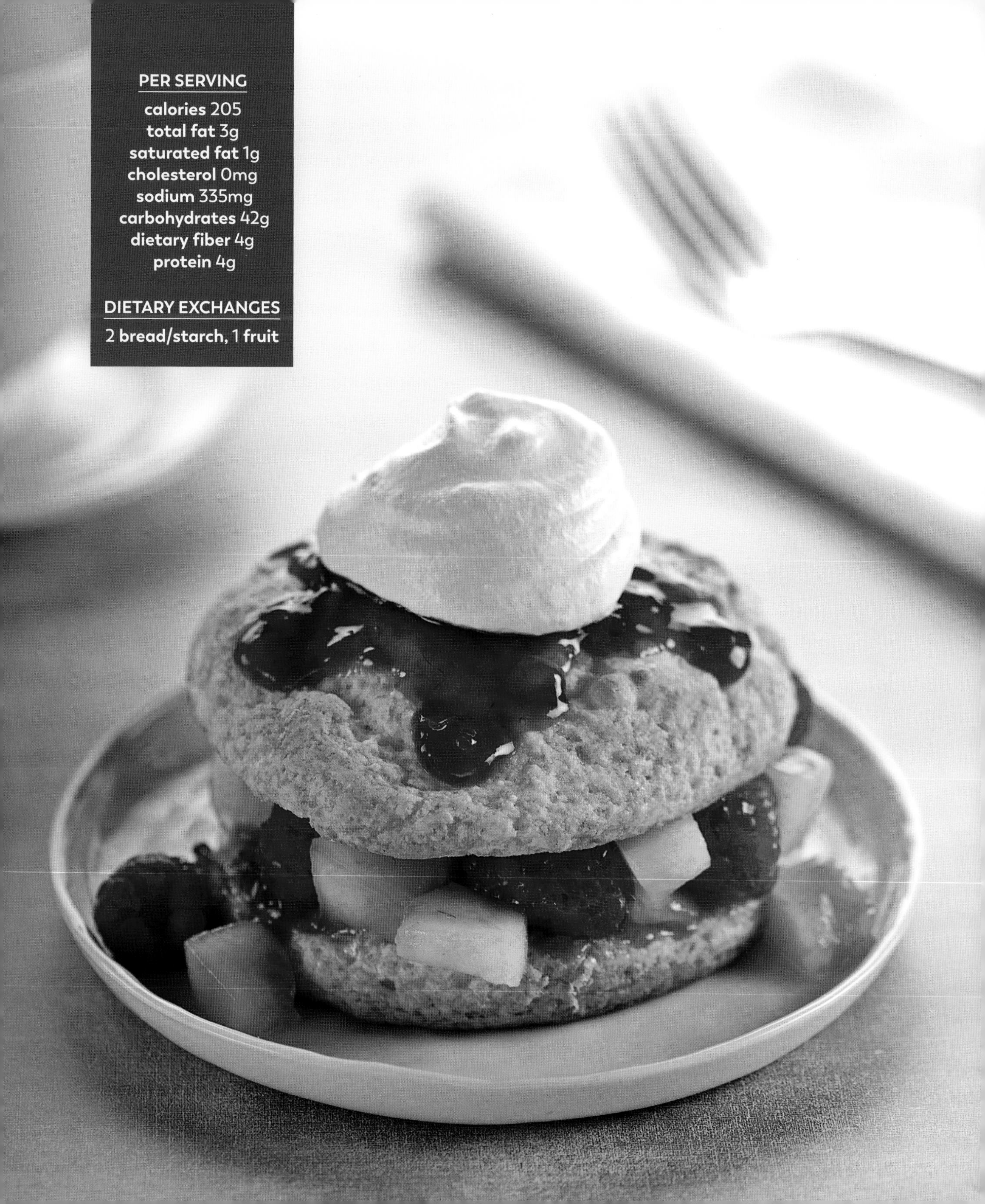

delicious desserts

Peach-Melba Shortcakes

Makes 4 servings

1 cup reduced-fat biscuit baking mix

¼ cup fat-free (skim) milk

2 tablespoons sugar

1¼ cups fresh raspberries

1 cup diced peeled peaches

2 tablespoons raspberry fruit spread

4 tablespoons thawed frozen whipped topping

1. Preheat oven to 425°F. Stir baking mix, milk and sugar in small bowl until smooth and well blended. Drop about 3 tablespoons per biscuit onto ungreased baking sheet. Bake 10 to 12 minutes or until tops are slightly browned. Cool on baking sheet 5 minutes.

2. Meanwhile, combine raspberries and peaches in medium bowl; set aside.

3. Microwave fruit spread in small microwavable bowl on HIGH 15 seconds or until softened.

4. Slice warm biscuits in half. Arrange biscuit bottoms on four serving plates. Drizzle ½ teaspoon fruit spread over each biscuit bottom. Top evenly with raspberries and peaches. Replace biscuit tops. Drizzle each shortcake with 1 teaspoon fruit spread; top with 1 tablespoon whipped topping.

Over the Rainbow

Makes 3 servings

1½ **cups orange juice**

⅓ **cup rainbow sherbet**

½ **cup club soda**

Additional rainbow sherbet for garnish (optional)

1. Combine orange juice and sherbet in blender. Process until smooth. Pour into glasses; add club soda.

2. Top with additional sherbet, if desired.

PER SERVING
calories 85
total fat 0g
saturated fat 0g
cholesterol 1mg
sodium 60mg
carbohydrates 20g
dietary fiber 0g
protein 0g

DIETARY EXCHANGES
1 fruit

Fruit Salad with Creamy Banana Dressing

Makes 8 servings

2 cups fresh pineapple chunks

1 cup cantaloupe cubes

1 cup honeydew melon cubes

1 cup fresh blackberries

1 cup sliced fresh strawberries

1 cup seedless red grapes

1 medium apple, diced

2 medium ripe bananas, sliced

½ cup vanilla nonfat Greek yogurt

2 tablespoons honey

1 tablespoon fresh lemon juice

¼ teaspoon ground nutmeg

1. Combine pineapple, cantaloupe, honeydew, blackberries, strawberries, grapes and apple in large bowl; mix gently.

2. Combine bananas, yogurt, honey, lemon juice and nutmeg in blender or food processor; blend until smooth.

3. Pour dressing over fruit mixture; gently toss to coat. Serve immediately.

PER SERVING
calories 125
total fat 0g
saturated fat 0g
cholesterol 0mg
sodium 15mg
carbohydrates 31g
dietary fiber 4g
protein 3g

DIETARY EXCHANGES
2 fruit

Mug-Made Mocha Cake

Makes 1 serving

2 tablespoons whole wheat flour

2 tablespoons sugar

1 tablespoon cocoa powder, plus
   additional for garnish

1½ to 2 teaspoons instant coffee
   granules

1 egg white

3 tablespoons fat-free (skim) milk

1 teaspoon vegetable oil

2 teaspoons mini semisweet
   chocolate chips

1 tablespoon thawed frozen
   fat-free whipped topping

Microwave Directions

1. Combine flour, sugar, 1 tablespoon cocoa and coffee granules in large ceramic* microwavable mug; mix well. Whisk egg white, milk and oil in small bowl until well blended. Stir into flour mixture until smooth. Fold in chocolate chips.

2. Microwave on HIGH 2 minutes. Let stand 1 to 2 minutes before serving. Top with whipped topping and additional cocoa, if desired.

This cake will only work in a ceramic mug as the material allows for more even cooking than glass.

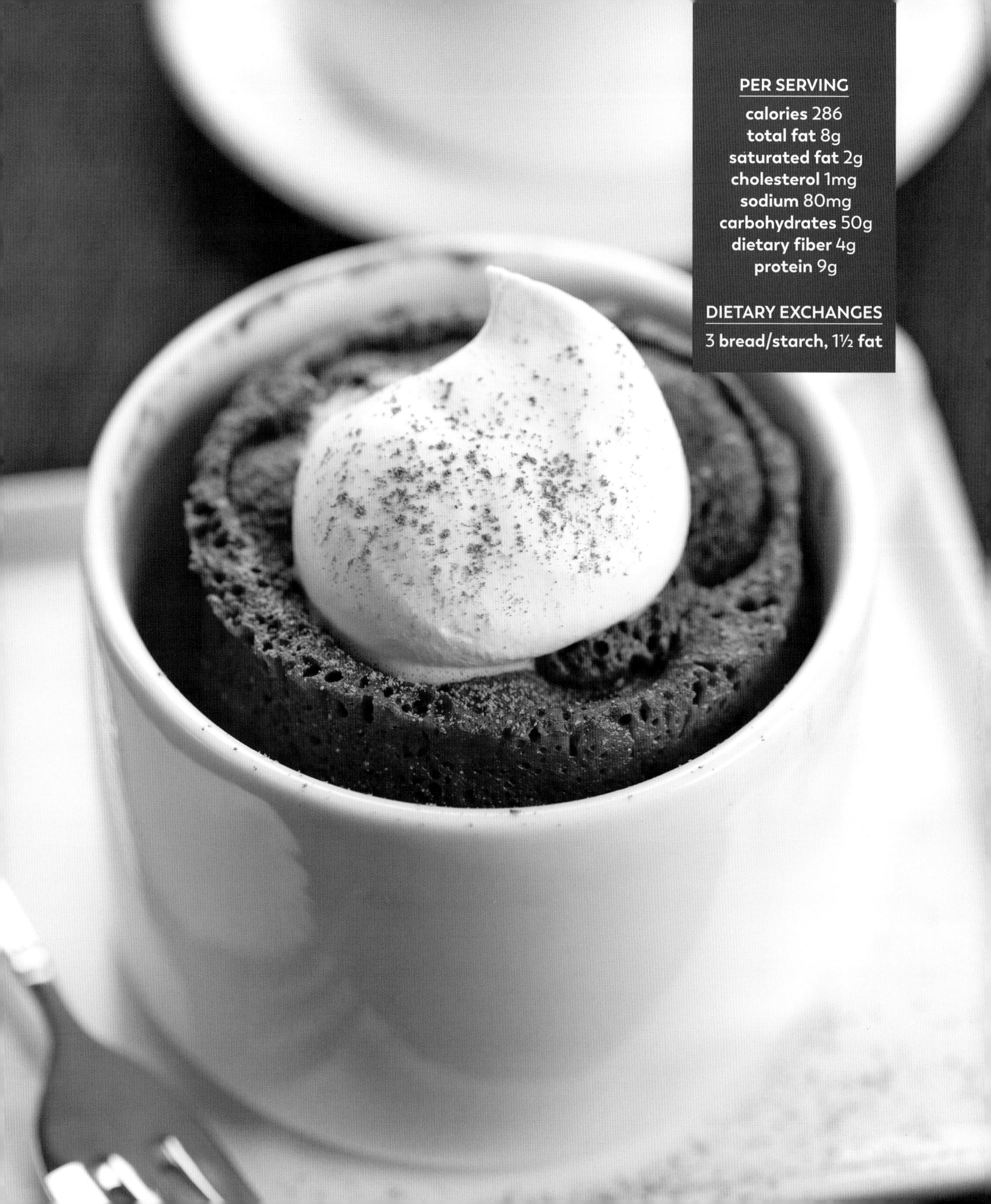

PER SERVING

calories 286
total fat 8g
saturated fat 2g
cholesterol 1mg
sodium 80mg
carbohydrates 50g
dietary fiber 4g
protein 9g

DIETARY EXCHANGES

3 **bread/starch,** 1½ **fat**

Peppermint-Chip Cake in a Cup

Makes 1 serving

¼ cup angel food cake mix

3 tablespoons water

1 tablespoon mini semisweet chocolate chips, plus additional for garnish

2 tablespoons thawed frozen fat-free whipped topping

⅛ teaspoon peppermint extract

Crushed peppermints* (optional)

*To crush peppermints, place unwrapped candy in a heavy-duty resealable food storage bag. Loosely seal the bag, leaving an opening for air to escape. Crush the candies thoroughly with a rolling pin, meat mallet or the bottom of a heavy skillet.

Microwave Directions

1. Combine cake mix, water and 1 tablespoon chocolate chips in large ceramic** microwavable mug.

2. Microwave on HIGH 1½ minutes. Let stand 1 to 2 minutes.

3. Meanwhile, stir whipped topping and peppermint extract in small bowl until well blended. Spoon over cake. Top with additional chocolate chips and crushed peppermints, if desired. Serve immediately.

**This cake will only work in a ceramic mug as the material allows for more even cooking than glass.

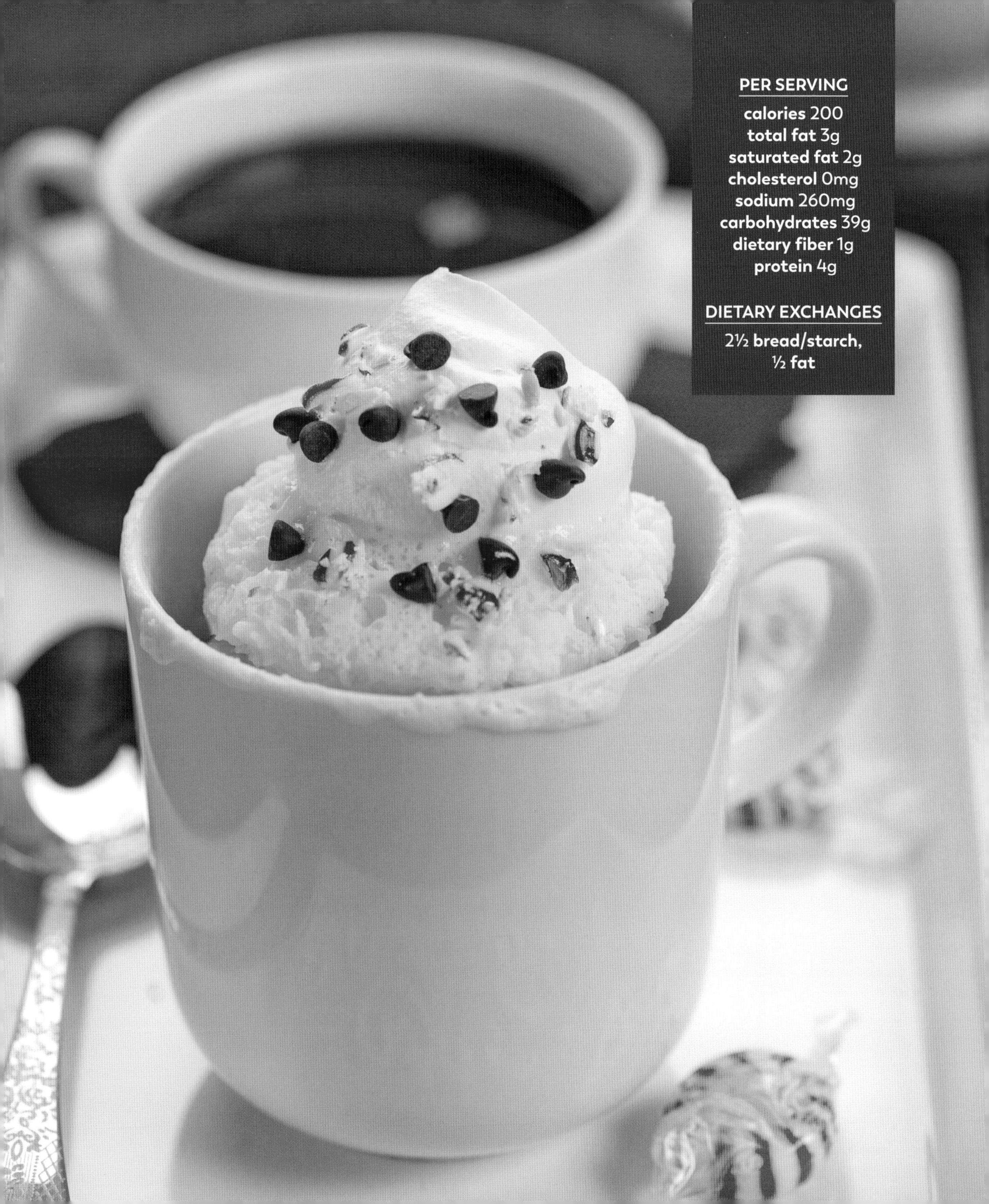

PER SERVING

calories 200
total fat 3g
saturated fat 2g
cholesterol 0mg
sodium 260mg
carbohydrates 39g
dietary fiber 1g
protein 4g

DIETARY EXCHANGES

2½ **bread/starch,**
½ **fat**

Grilled Peaches with Spicy Cream Cheese Topping

Makes 6 servings

½ cup (4 ounces) light cream cheese, softened

1 tablespoon honey

¼ teaspoon ground red pepper

2 cups thawed frozen fat-free whipped topping

6 peaches, halved and pitted

¼ cup slivered almonds, toasted*

Fresh mint leaves (optional)

*To toast almonds, spread in single layer in heavy skillet. Cook and stir over medium heat 1 to 2 minutes or until nuts are lightly browned, stirring frequently.

1. Prepare grill for direct cooking over medium-high heat. Spray grid with nonstick cooking spray.

2. Gently stir cream cheese in medium bowl until smooth. Whisk in honey and ground red pepper until well blended. Fold in whipped topping. Cover and refrigerate until ready to use.

3. Place peaches, cut sides down, on prepared grill. Grill, covered, 2 to 3 minutes. Turn over; grill 2 to 3 minutes or until peaches begin to soften. Remove to plate; let stand to cool slightly.

4. Arrange 2 peach halves, cut sides up, on six serving plates. Top evenly with spicy cream cheese topping and almonds. Garnish with mint.

PER SERVING
calories 182
total fat 6g
saturated fat 2g
cholesterol 13mg
sodium 107mg
carbohydrates 28g
dietary fiber 3g
protein 4g

DIETARY EXCHANGES
1 bread/starch,
1 fruit, 1 fat

Strawberry Cheesecake Parfaits

Makes 4 servings

1½ cups vanilla nonfat Greek yogurt

½ cup whipped cream cheese, at room temperature

2 tablespoons powdered sugar

1 teaspoon vanilla

2 cups sliced fresh strawberries

2 teaspoons granulated sugar

8 honey graham cracker squares, coarsely crumbled (about 2 cups)

Fresh mint leaves (optional)

1. Whisk yogurt, cream cheese, powdered sugar and vanilla in small bowl until smooth and well blended.

2. Combine strawberries and granulated sugar in small bowl; gently toss.

3. Layer ¼ cup yogurt mixture, ¼ cup strawberries and ¼ cup graham cracker crumbs in each of four dessert dishes. Repeat layers. Garnish with mint. Serve immediately.

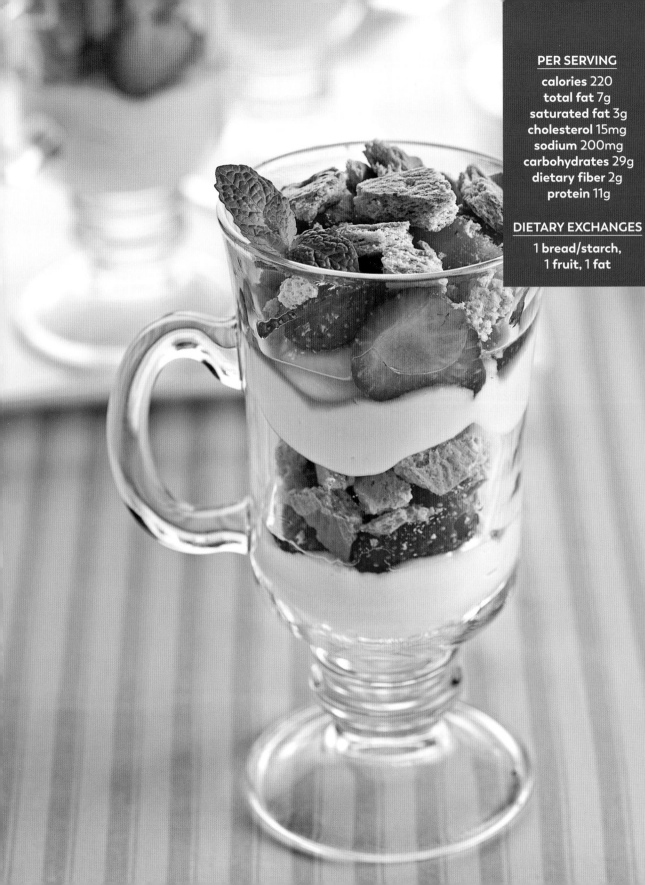

PER SERVING
calories 220
total fat 7g
saturated fat 3g
cholesterol 15mg
sodium 200mg
carbohydrates 29g
dietary fiber 2g
protein 11g

DIETARY EXCHANGES
1 bread/starch,
1 fruit, 1 fat

Creamy Banana Parfait with Nutmeg

Makes 4 servings

1 container (6 ounces) vanilla nonfat yogurt

2 ounces reduced-fat cream cheese, softened

1¼ cups fat-free (skim) milk

¼ teaspoon vanilla

1 package (4-serving size) sugar-free instant vanilla pudding and pie filling mix

⅛ teaspoon ground nutmeg

1 ripe medium banana, very thinly sliced

12 low-fat vanilla wafers, crushed (about ½ cup)

¼ cup thawed frozen fat-free whipped topping

1. Combine yogurt and cream cheese in medium bowl; beat with electric mixer at medium speed until smooth. Gradually add milk and vanilla; beat until smooth. Add pudding mix and nutmeg; beat until well blended.

2. Spoon pudding mixture into each of four wine goblets or parfait glasses. Top with banana slices; sprinkle with cookie crumbs. (Cover bananas evenly with cookie crumbs to prevent discoloration.)

3. Cover parfaits with plastic wrap. Refrigerate at least 1 hour or up to 4 hours before serving.

4. Top each parfait with 2 tablespoons whipped topping.

Tropical Parfait

Makes 4 servings

1½ cups orange or vanilla nonfat yogurt

1 can (11 ounces) mandarin orange segments in light syrup, drained and chopped

1 can (8 ounces) pineapple chunks in juice, drained

1 medium banana, sliced

2 tablespoons shredded coconut, toasted*

*To toast coconut, spread in single layer in heavy-bottomed skillet. Cook and stir over medium heat 1 to 2 minutes or until lightly browned. Remove from skillet immediately. Cool before using.

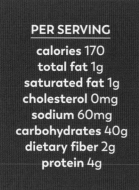

PER SERVING
calories 170
total fat 1g
saturated fat 1g
cholesterol 0mg
sodium 60mg
carbohydrates 40g
dietary fiber 2g
protein 4g

DIETARY EXCHANGES
1 bread/starch, 2 fruit

1. Combine yogurt and oranges in medium bowl; mix well.

2. Spoon half of yogurt mixture into four serving bowls; top with pineapple. Spoon remaining yogurt mixture over pineapple; top with banana slices. Sprinkle with coconut. Serve immediately.

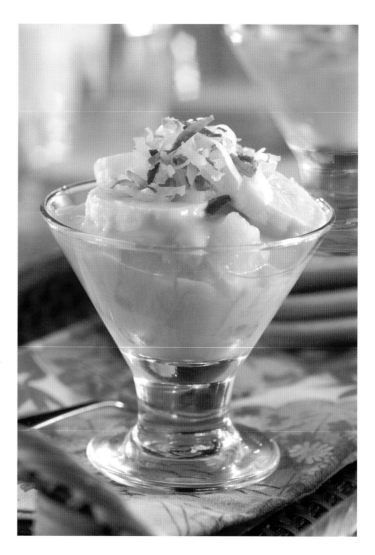

index

Metric Conversion Chart

VOLUME MEASUREMENTS (dry)

$\frac{1}{8}$ teaspoon = 0.5 mL
$\frac{1}{4}$ teaspoon = 1 mL
$\frac{1}{2}$ teaspoon = 2 mL
$\frac{3}{4}$ teaspoon = 4 mL
1 teaspoon = 5 mL
1 tablespoon = 15 mL
2 tablespoons = 30 mL
$\frac{1}{4}$ cup = 60 mL
$\frac{1}{3}$ cup = 75 mL
$\frac{1}{2}$ cup = 125 mL
$\frac{2}{3}$ cup = 150 mL
$\frac{3}{4}$ cup = 175 mL
1 cup = 250 mL
2 cups = 1 pint = 500 mL
3 cups = 750 mL
4 cups = 1 quart = 1 L

VOLUME MEASUREMENTS (fluid)

1 fluid ounce (2 tablespoons) = 30 mL
4 fluid ounces ($\frac{1}{2}$ cup) = 125 mL
8 fluid ounces (1 cup) = 250 mL
12 fluid ounces ($1\frac{1}{2}$ cups) = 375 mL
16 fluid ounces (2 cups) = 500 mL

WEIGHTS (mass)

$\frac{1}{2}$ ounce = 15 g
1 ounce = 30 g
3 ounces = 90 g
4 ounces = 120 g
8 ounces = 225 g
10 ounces = 285 g
12 ounces = 360 g
16 ounces = 1 pound = 450 g

DIMENSIONS

$\frac{1}{16}$ inch = 2 mm
$\frac{1}{8}$ inch = 3 mm
$\frac{1}{4}$ inch = 6 mm
$\frac{1}{2}$ inch = 1.5 cm
$\frac{3}{4}$ inch = 2 cm
1 inch = 2.5 cm

OVEN TEMPERATURES

250°F = 120°C
275°F = 140°C
300°F = 150°C
325°F = 160°C
350°F = 180°C
375°F = 190°C
400°F = 200°C
425°F = 220°C
450°F = 230°C

BAKING PAN SIZES

Utensil	Size in Inches/Quarts	Metric Volume	Size in Centimeters
Baking or Cake Pan (square or rectangular)	8×8×2	2 L	20×20×5
	9×9×2	2.5 L	23×23×5
	12×8×2	3 L	30×20×5
	13×9×2	3.5 L	33×23×5
Loaf Pan	8×4×3	1.5 L	20×10×7
	9×5×3	2 L	23×13×7
Round Layer Cake Pan	8×1½	1.2 L	20×4
	9×1½	1.5 L	23×4
Pie Plate	8×1¼	750 mL	20×3
	9×1¼	1 L	23×3
Baking Dish or Casserole	1 quart	1 L	—
	1½ quart	1.5 L	—
	2 quart	2 L	—